YOUR BIRTHRIGHT:

EXCEPTIONAL
HEALTH AND VITALITY

by Milorad Masic

Published by Milorad Masic

For information e-mail inquiries at:
miloradmagic@yahoo.com

Text and art copyright © 2007.

Printed in United Kingdom

ISBN: 978–0–9556605–0–4

DEDICATION

To all the truth-seekers who encouraged me to persevere, see the light at the end of the tunnel and share my message with them: this book is affectionately dedicated to you!

The Author

"If you face the fact,
it becomes the truth;
if you escape,
you live in lies."

(Heraclitus)

ೲഐ

"Truth is incontrovertible;
malice may attack it,
ignorance may deride it,
but in the end there it is."

(Winston Churchill)

CONTENTS

LEGAL EXCLUSION CLAUSE OF THE ANOTHER KIND

As we live in an increasingly litigious society – a society overburdened by various authorities – it has become virtually requisite for health related books to carry a legal exclusion clause. Most of the exclusion clauses that I have seen, and probably you too will have read some of them before, imply that the material presented in the book in question is not intended as a substitute for the advice of a qualified doctor. Those exclusion clauses go on to advise that you consult a physician before putting into practice any suggestions those books have set out. And they invariably end with the author and the publisher excluding all liability for any adverse consequences resulting from following the practical guiding principles outlined in their book.

This book is intended to take the above approach to a higher plane. You should not read this book unless and until you are prepared to accept personal primary responsibility for your own health and vitality. The aim of this book is to awaken you from cultural hypnosis, broaden your horizons and make you aware that you must be proactive in your own health and vitality. Health care should not be delegated to any expert and anybody reading this book must be able to evaluate any advice given by a physician for himself or herself without blindly accepting it. The same is true for the contents of this book. The "buck" must begin and stop with you, as yours is the final judgment, as yours is the ultimate authority. Any exclusion clause that proposes otherwise does everyone a great disservice.

With the mantle firmly in your hands, I challenge you to decide whether to read on. And remember, whatever your decision is, it will shape your destiny. So, choose well!

ACKNOWLEDGMENTS

The information presented in this book is the result of several years personal research triggered by my own illness, by my frustration with doctors and their inability to truly help me to regain my health, as well as my frustration with myself for blindly following them. At the end of the day, it was the miracle-work of love that turned the tide around and guided me magically to reclaim my birthright.

For these intense lessons, drawn from my own experience, to come to light in the form of this book, there is a lineage of giants of people to whom I am truly grateful for giving me expansive perspective. The list is too long to mention them all here. Therefore, I would like to acknowledge and give a special praising to the following individuals who have influenced me most:

My mother who, like only the exceptional mothers do, showers her children with understanding, compassion and warmth. Her unconditional love and support have profoundly shaped my life philosophy, and her inspiring example is constantly reminding me of the power of love, active faith, patience, persistence, and the notion that nothing in life is impossible once you accept responsibility and get committed. You are the true giant in my life.

My sunshine – my leading lady, who with her gracious attention and care helped me align my consciousness with my heart and make a quantum leap on my quest for wellness. Your love gives me the strength and the peace of mind to create. I adore you, honey.

My bohemian friend and artist Branko Simic, who produced the mind-boggling and profoundly inspiring illustrations for this book. It has been said that each picture is worth a thousand words. These illustrations are worth much more – they bring vibrant luminosity to the book. No words can express their true worth – for only their appreciation can do that.

My dear friend Anthony Grey, the best-selling author of novels "Saigon" and "Peking", who encouraged me to write this book, read and commented upon the entire manuscript, and enthusiastically advised me on its presentation. I deeply value our friendship.

I am very grateful to Robyn Wilson, a prominent entrepreneur and writer, for proofreading the manuscript, as well as for her insights and understanding. Thank you for being a light.

In addition, I hereby wish to express my gratitude to those who granted permission for the following material to be quoted:

1. From "How to Read a Book", revised edition, by Mortimer J. Adler and Charles Van Doren. Copyright 1940, and renewed © 1967, by Mortimer J. Adler. Copyright © 1972 by Mortimer J. Adler and Charles Van Doren. Reprinted by permission of Simon & Schuster Adult Publishing Group.

2. From "Dr Zhivago" by Boris Pasternak, published by Harvill Press. Reprinted by permission of The Random House Group Ltd.

3. From "The Treasury of Quotes" by Jim Rohn, published by Health Communications, Inc. Reprinted by permission of Jim Rohn International.

4. From "Quantum Healing" by Deepak Chopra, published by Bantam Books. Reprinted by permission of Random House, Inc.

And to everyone else who has been on my side in the dance of life – you know who you are – I salute you.

FOREWORD
by Anthony Grey

I read this short powerful book in two and a half hours. Its brevity and succinctness make it particularly effective and memorable.

At heart it is the story of the author's own voyage of self discovery at a relatively young age through the rough seas of his own painful and potentially disabling illness for which conventional medicine could offer no cure. His greatest realisation eventually was that it was up to him – and indeed to every one of us – to accept or reject the conventional treatment we are offered and take total responsibility for our own health and wellbeing.

The resultant detective work that enabled Milorad to become well again led him to vital discoveries about our natural energies and strengths which can warrant our own salvation if we are wise enough to apply them. Milorad tells the story of his own suffering very briefly and passingly and focuses with inspiring freshness on the fundamental principles which his experience indicates can ensure the good workings of our physical bodies and minds. So fundamental are these understandings, he says, that they should be regarded as the common birthright of us all.

I met Milorad some ten years ago in 1997 at a self-development seminar and have known him through much of his time of suffering and recovery. His appearance during most of that time, gaunt and underweight reflected his battle with his interconnected maladies. Today, however, as this book goes to press in early 2007 his appearance has become that of a glowingly healthy man looking younger than at any time since I have known him and this fact alone is a testimonial to his story and his determined search for solutions to what at times were near-crippling pain and disability.

A courageous, determined and resourceful individual Milorad has produced a book capable of encouraging and re-inspiring us all to follow his example and learn to overcome the many fierce health challenges of modern life. Consequently I heartily commend this uniquely brief health book to all who wish to follow Milorad's example and reclaim their birthright by uncompromisingly taking ultimate responsibility for their own health into their own hands.

Spring 2007
Norwich, England

Anthony Grey is the international best-selling author of the novels "Saigon", "Peking" and "Tokyo Bay" and most recently the 2007 autobiographical memoir "The Thoughts of Chairman Grey"

Preface

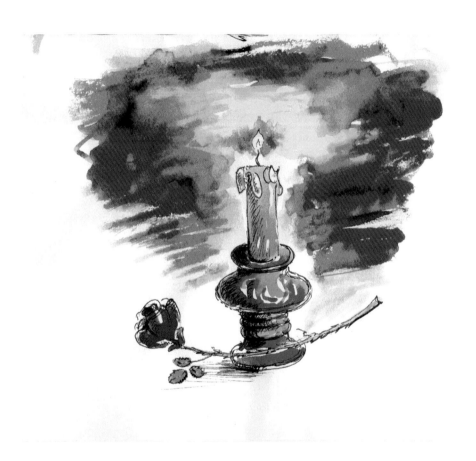

"Love yourself and watch - today,
tomorrow, always."
(Gautama the Buddha)

*"Doctors pour drugs of which they know little,
to cure diseases of which they know less,
into human beings of whom they know nothing."*

(Voltaire)

PREFACE

"Doctors pour drugs of which they know little, to cure diseases of which they know less, into human beings of whom they know nothing." (Voltaire)

Several years ago I almost became another number in the statistics of medical accidents. I had been taking painkillers to "cure" my Ankylosing Spondylitis – the severest form of arthritis – for several years. Yes, you've read it correctly, for several years. My doctor assured me that it was okay and that my body was coping well with them. But I did not know that whilst those painkillers were easing the pain in my joints somewhat, they were at the same time blocking my body's absorption of ascorbic acid (vitamin C), which is essential for the production of cartilage – the connective tissue surrounding the joints. Thus these painkillers were in fact working against my body's ability to combat the connective tissue breakdown, which was the very cause of my condition. I should have known better.

I suppose the doctors were just doing their job to the best of their ability under the given circumstance of overwhelming workload. Or, was it a part of the widespread cunning conspiracy aimed at controlling and reducing the world population? I do not know. But, what was I doing? Well... to be frank, I was blindly following the "higher" authority. For several years?! I am afraid so. And then the disaster struck. My stomach collapsed and gave up. I almost died. Would blaming the medical profession have helped me? No, not at all. Could some other doctor have helped? Not likely. My experience mirrored the thoughts and beliefs that I had then. I had to change, and change quickly. I had to open up to the new level of wisdom within me. And I did. I did it resolutely and wholeheartedly. *"The heart has its reasons that the reason cannot know,"* the famous aphorism of Blaise Pascal has it.

13

The human spirit has the power to rise above all odds. That is why you are reading these lines now. They come from my heart. Even though I am still traversing tirelessly on this newly discovered path and see this journey as a never-ending learning quest, I feel deeply with all of you who can relate to this story in any way. Nobody else ought to suffer the way I did.

Recent scientific research has revealed that medical "accidents" cause far more deaths annually (98,000) than car accidents (43,000), breast cancer (42,000) or AIDS (16,000) in the USA. Medical error deaths are the same as if three "jumbo-jets", full of passengers on board, were to crash down every day. Prescription drugs kill more Britons (70,000) than cancer. According to data published by the World Health Organisation, global death toll caused by AIDS is circa 40,000 while that from medicaments is staggering 700,000 people annually. I believe that the actual numbers are much greater as the above represent only the officially recorded cases.

The medical profession is increasingly preoccupied with the tendency to treat lifestyle problems as diseases. In this process the focus is on the consequences of these lifestyle problems rather than on the actual causes of the problems.

"A plant can live without its blossoms but not without its roots," said an ancient Chinese sage. Our health care system has truly become a disease care system. This very trend has lead to the increasing medicalisation of society and, consequently to those horrifying statistics listed above.

Doctors and, above all, pharmaceutical companies are being blamed for the excessive medicalisation. Their disease-mongering is often seen as a way to expand markets for new products. "Great advances" of medicine are being vociferously presented to us, while nothing is being said about their adverse side effects. Moreover, medicaments only serve to suppress symptoms. The suppression of symptoms of illness without regard to the basic cause of the symptoms is shallow.

Sadly, this ignorance is widespread. By saying this I do not intend to undermine the importance of modern medicine, especially when it comes to cases of accidents and emergency. <u>My purpose and my mission here is to awaken you</u> – to get the message out and have you tune in, to inform you, to expand your awareness and empower you to take charge of your health and vitality.

Nowadays, we are constantly being bombarded with advertisements for various over-the-counter pain-killing drugs, especially via the medium of television. We are being subliminally indoctrinated into the morbid belief that the pain is the ultimate evil which is to be banished quickly with medications, ignoring the fact that the best way to eliminate pain is to eliminate the abuse of natural laws of life. Those ideas thus become unexamined habits of mind which thwart effective living instead of aiding it. Is it surprising than that more and more people fear pain more than they fear death? And really, you should not fear either.

And how about recent hypocritical warnings from European Union government's agencies against taking vitamins without prescriptions while nothing is being done to control sales of other over-the-counter medications that do us more harm than good?

It seems that the commercial market place and the importance of corporate profits define more and more of our lives. Even health, the most sacred of human values, is for sale. If they are really concerned about the well-being of the population, then officials should think about <u>making the study of health and vitality a part of the school curriculum</u>.

According to German philosopher Otto Weininger, the afore mentioned trends in medicine are largely due to the Jewish liking for Chemistry and the influence of the Jews in world affairs. And, he himself was a Jew.

So what else can one do? You will have heard about the alternative medicine methods. I will not tell you anything about them. There are scores of qualified people who could do that much better than I could do it. I am here to talk about **you** and what you can do for yourselves and your well-being.

Health and vitality are the very foundation of your happiness in life. When you are healthy and vital you can achieve everything, and if you are not then it is difficult to enjoy the life to the full and be happy. The focus of this book is on the aspects of our lives that greatly affect our health and vitality. I want to share with you some insights concerning life and health drawn from my own health challenges, some common sense practical guidelines that have improved my health and vitality far beyond what the doctors told me that I should expect. You may want to apply them in your life for, say, a few weeks and see for yourself what difference occurs.

The will to live happily is extraordinarily potent and our focused mind can lead to the transformation of our lives. It gives rise to the vital brain impulses that in turn activate your endocrine system and create "miracles". That connection between faith and the will to live enables the body to rise to any challenge. You only need to accept that something can be done about any challenge to your health and vitality, and such a belief will lead you far beyond the boundaries of possibilities set by medical profession. And then, if you decide to go back to the "old ways" – be my guest. An old proverb has it that your body is the temple of your soul. And then it goes on to urge us to treat our body like a temple, as it is the only place we have to live in.

This book is packed with real, concise facts of life that will help you understand how to improve your health and vitality. It is jargon-free, so you do not need to have a degree in medicine to understand it. Neither do you need to have any previous knowledge about the subject in order to come to grip with these empowering, life-changing insights. And then it will be up to you to have the discipline – discipline born out of awareness and understanding – to consistently apply the simple guiding principles I write about, and succeed.

May the forthcoming pages provide all of you who read them with the awareness and inspiration that will lead you back to yourselves and empower you to embark on the road to exceptional health and vitality!

Chapter One

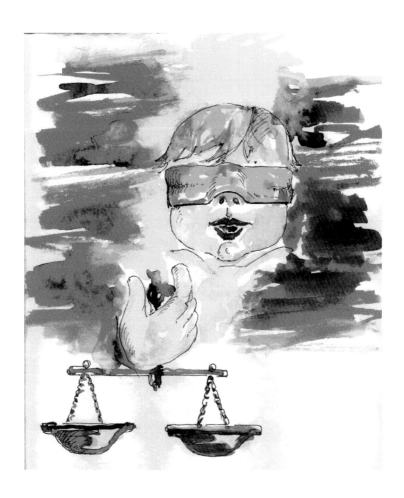

Personal Responsibility

*"Nothing splendid has ever been achieved,
except by those who dared believe
that something inside of them
was superior to circumstance."*

(Bruce Barton)

PERSONAL RESPONSIBILITY

"Nothing splendid has ever been achieved, except by those who dared believe that something inside of them was superior to circumstance." (Bruce Barton)

When asked the question: "What is most important to you in your life?" majority would answer with "Health!" And yet a great many people have some kind of health challenge nowadays. So, what is going on here? Why do those two facts contradict one another so significantly? Most people tend to take their health for granted, until they lose it at least. And that is precisely what had happened to me.

This era in which we live brings big life-style changes on a daily basis. We adjust our lives to those changes and demands. Often, we find ourselves caught in situations and activities which do not serve our purpose best. Along the way, we regard the matters that are urgent as important and the things that are truly important we take as less urgent. Stress takes over, our nerves are tense, we do not eat regularly, we exercise less and less, and we neglect ourselves and our loved ones. This pattern becomes a habit that goes on day after day after day, ad infinitum. And when we act habitually, our awareness is at its lowest point. One day we wake up with realisation that we are where we do not want to be, or that we are where we want to be, but we do not enjoy the process. We feel that life is eluding us, a sense of emptiness overwhelms us and many of us become overweight, lose our nerves and succumb to various illnesses as result. Sounds familiar, doesn't it. Well, here is where the old saying goes: *"For things to get better, you have to get better; for things to change, you have to change…"*.

The great majority of people are not prepared to change. For them those challenges are someone else's responsibility and someone else should sort them out. How many times have you heard people say: "Doctor knows the best."? Well, I find it difficult to buy this one. By blindly accepting and following opinion of the external "authority", you may endanger your life, just as I did. Your doctor should be your friend, someone who pays attention to what you have to say, someone who cares sincerely and someone who you can listen to with trust and confidence. But, the ultimate expert for you is you, as you are health-wise where you are today from the choices, decisions and actions you have made. And, if you have on some level generated your health challenges, you can change the situation around if you do not like it. No one else is responsible. If you believe that you create your world, then take charge of your health and your life and change. It is the little changes in your life-style that make the big difference in your health and vitality. Please remember, the worst form of insanity is doing the same thing over and over again and expecting a different outcome. Get rid of the belief that someone else is responsible, since when someone else is responsible then you cannot change, because the change then has to come through that someone else, and that in itself is overly second grade and out of place. When you give your responsibility away, you give away your self-respect and with it your love for your being and ultimately your freedom. And remember: freedom is the basic requirement for your soul to grow.

This book is about you – responsible you. Taking personal responsibility for your health and vitality will transform your life forever. The most important step on that journey is to take charge of the actual underlying cause of your health challenges. Nowadays doctors prescribe drugs that suppress symptoms, but do not remove the cause of disease. For the sake of quick relief on one hand and huge profits that the prescription drugs bring to the pharmaceutical corporations on the other, many unnecessary and harmful "reliefs" are being administered. If given treatment does not remove the cause of disease, it does not either cure or prevent it. Please, reclaim responsibility for your well-being, from which your culture and society have alienated you. It is your responsibility. It is your right. *"Rights never stand alone; they always entail responsibilities,"* supposed Dr Pierce. In fact, this right and this responsibility are two sides of the same entity – you.

In order to build and maintain our health and vitality we need to responsibly observe a way of living that is presented to us all by Mother Nature. These laws are imprinted into us all. **Quality of your health and vitality, and your life, is a matter of your relationships to sunlight, air, water, food, the environment, the people around you, and yourself.** Be truly aware of them, of their interdependence and their interplay, as well as of your role in the process. Your personal responsibility entails responding and relating to these factors truthfully – acting out of the present moment awareness, rather than reacting to them out of your old habits. And, responding to them truthfully and accepting the consequences of your actions without any complaint means being responsible. Your life is intimately connected with Nature. Nature is in a deep harmony. How about you? To abuse these essential agents of life is to abuse your own being. To even think that you can live against the laws of Nature and get away with it is a grand illusion. Your violation of those fundamental laws is what brings a galore of ailments upon you and what ultimately destroys you. So much for the deluded perceptions.

Awareness, understanding and personal responsibility are related to personal power – your ability to resolutely take the right course of action and to do consistently so. Along with the gift of consciousness comes your freedom to choose whether to act in harmony with Nature or not. And out of that freedom comes your responsibility. I urge you to be true, to be honest to yourself – there is no greater responsibility than that. Your old attitudes need to die and new ones need to be born. **You** have to bring about new values – values of truthfulness, sincerity and self-respect – into your life. Your health and vitality deserve the highest priority.

In the forthcoming chapters you will be shown what you can do for yourself in order to expand on what you are capable of and to turn around any challenging experience. Every chapter brings some new perspectives, new insights that will dissolve some old imprint in your memory by making you see things in a new light and empower you to find answers for yourselves. Like your friend, or a family member, or a doctor, I intend to be your inspiration and your guide to creating a profound change in your health and vitality, including the reversal of many challenging conditions caused by inadequate patterns and habits. Ultimately, it will be you putting up the effort and doing the work. You have to give these things to yourself.

My own experience, my inner journey, my inner experience of growing awareness, understanding and responsibility, and what I have learned from it and because of it, is what I am eager to share with you here. The biggest lesson life has taught me is that if you have a compelling reason and if you care enough about a result, you will act responsibly – with an open mind and open heart – and without a shadow of doubt you will attain it. By simply changing your perceptions, by allowing yourself to be guided by your awareness of the truth, you can change your life. Be honest with yourself while you journey through this book and through your life. *"Freedom is the will to be responsible to ourselves,"* said Fredrich Nietzche.

Be responsible for everything that you are and everything that you want to become. Your feelings of sincerity and responsibility will take you where your heart has always longed to go – to the royal road to vigorous health and vitality.

Please remember this simple truth: <u>The most important person in your life is you!</u>

Chapter Two

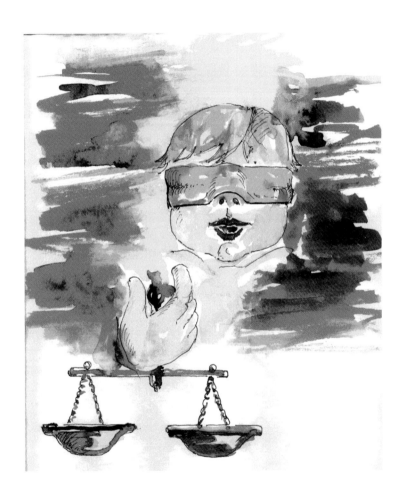

Energy – The Essence Of Life

*"The myriad of ailments all begin with energy.
The moment there is energy imbalance,
any ailment might occur."*

(Yellow Emperor)

ENERGY – THE ESSENCE OF LIFE

"The myriad of ailments all begin with energy. The moment there is energy imbalance, any ailment might occur." (Yellow Emperor)

One of the greatest lessons that I learned from my experience with arthritis was the realisation of what we humans truly are. My physical body was aching, or at least that's what my senses were telling me. Yet, I knew I was more than just a physical body. How did I know that? My mind was telling me so. But, my mind could tell me only that what it had absorbed during my lifetime. As that knowledge had existed before my birth, I concluded I wasn't my mind either. Then I realised there is that without which my body would be still, that without which my mind would simply evaporate, that without which my soul would wither, that without which there would be no life. That catalyst, which sustains it all – our bodies, our minds, our souls, our lives and existence of everything around us, is the same force – energy.

The energy that flows through your body is only a tiny fraction of the energy of Nature, and the energy of the Universe. In fact, there is no energy in your body other than that derived from the interlocking, ambient force field of Nature – from the wheelwork of the Universe. Your life is intimately connected with Nature. How well you accommodate and adapt to the laws of Nature will determine how well you draw upon the spring of your life – energy. When you understand the usefulness of the energy and its universal laws, you will be able to utilise them effectively for the preservation of your health and vitality. Of the connectedness of vital energy or life force, with the vast field of energy of the universe, in the ancient Chinese classic "Tao Teh Ching", the sage Lao Tzu said beautifully: *"Present at every moment and ceaselessly continuing – this is the gateway to indescribable marvels."*

The human body is the greatest wonder on planet Earth. Its creation, development, functions and other processes are governed by the same life force – vital energy. It resides within and is distributed by our nervous system. Every atom of our body is 99.99% energy. This energy flows between the cells and organs and helps functioning of muscles, blood circulation, metabolism, immune system, thinking, replication of cells and other vital bodily functions. Without it life would be impossible. When energy is deficient our bodily functions get impaired and when it is abundant our bodies are healthy and vital.

Every day your body makes, on average, 10,000 steps, thinks 60,000 thoughts and pumps 35,000 litres of blood around your system. To meet all these requirements, your body requires energy. Energy flows through your body, along channels or "meridians", throughout your life. The stresses and strains of daily life tend to obstruct the free flow of energy and eventually to block it. Often we expend our energy faster than we recuperate it and with it we lower the functional efficiency of our bodies. Many people think that stimulants such as coffee, tea, refined sugar, cigarettes and alcohol can work as quick fixes when your energy levels are inadequate. In fact, they rob you of the very thing you need and also compromise your immune system. The very essential requirements for revival of our energies are rest, quiet and warmth.

We humans as well as all other living creatures are the power stations of Nature. With delicate sensitivity, we derive energy from sunlight, air, water and everything else that surrounds us, and we use it to sustain both our physical and mental faculties.

Energy comes through our cells. Hence, the quality of our life is fundamentally interconnected with the quality of life of our cells. Our bodies are made up of circa 75 trillion of cells. Every second approximately 5 million cells die and get immediately replaced with new ones. In order to function properly, and also to generate sufficient energy, our cells require oxygen, nutrients and ability to eliminate their metabolic waste. Everything taken in by our body has to be either assimilated or eliminated.

Due to a lifestyle, contemporary man needlessly and uselessly scatters and disperses his vital energy otherwise used for the normal metabolic processes. That leads to enervation, or fatigue if you prefer. The biochemistry of our bodies gets entangled and our minds become distorted. As a result, processes of secretion and excretion get impaired and toxins are retained. These toxins overstimulate and saturate the organism slightly below the point of active resistance, causing toleration to them, and finally they chronically poison the body. With the passage of time the flow of energy becomes compromised, metabolic waste piles up and, as a result, our bodies deteriorate. What is most concerning is the fact that the great majority of people are not even aware of it.

Our bodies are integrated systems made up of organs which are interdependent. The amount of energy that any organ can spend depends on finite bodily resources, as well as on the requirements of other organs. Should one part of the body draw extra energy in order to complete a desired task, there will be shortage in another part. For instance, one cannot run fast and solve a mathematical problem at the same time. This is governed by the natural low of compensation. An organ that overspends energy harms itself as well as the body as a whole. Our interference in the form of ignorant over-indulgences, triggered by the automatism of our minds and egos, is what leads to breakdown of energy balance and ultimately to breakdown of our bodies.

To bring back unity and harmony to our bodies we must first re-establish the balance of energy. The surest way of achieving that is by tuning into the power of our awareness, by developing new perceptions and by paying conscious attention to our bodily functions, instead of being on "automatic pilot". Both physical and psychological rest are required until the normal metabolism is restored, until toxins are eliminated and vital energy restored. At anytime, without any exception, when we exhaust our energy reservoir, rest is necessary for the recuperation of energy and the repair of the body. After the "batteries" are recharged and the unobstructed flow of energy is restored, a proper hygienic and dietetic lifestyle that does not create enervation should be followed, and consequently health and vitality will flourish.

In the chapters that follow you will be presented in more detail with the factors that affect your energy levels. My awareness of their influence, the recognition of the natural laws that govern them and my adherence to these principles have made a compelling difference in my energy department – from deficiency to abundance. I trust they could do the same for you.

Let's begin with...

Chapter Three

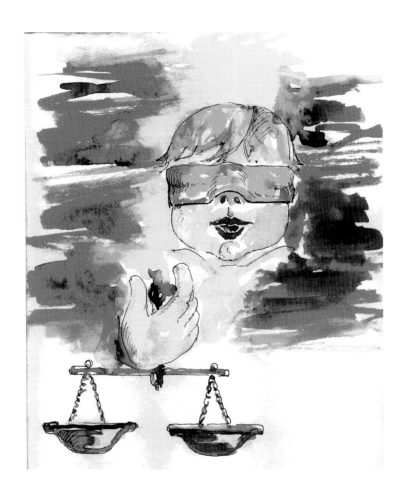

Sunlight Delight

"The feeling of health,
the full-noon trill,
the song of me rising from bed
and meeting the Sun."

(Walt Whitman)

SUNLIGHT DELIGHT

"The feeling of health, the full-noon trill, the song of me rising from bed and meeting the Sun." (Walt Whitman)

What an insight of Walt Whitman! And I agree with him one thousand percent. For some years now, I have been aiming to spend as much time as possible outdoors exposed to sunlight. To me, the benefits from such a practice have been immeasurable. My skin has become suppler, my bones have become stronger and my freshly illuminated spirit has set me off reaching for the infinite. Aren't you going to join the "club"? Hey, it is free!

The energising, modifying and developing powers of sunlight are neither sufficiently understood nor fully harnessed by us humans. Nevertheless, its powerful influence upon the functioning of living organisms is indisputable. Specific records about the importance of sunlight to humans date back to ancient Greece. Herodotus, who is considered to be the father of sunlight therapy said: *"Exposure to the sun is highly necessary in persons whose health needs restoring and who have need of putting on weight."*

The vital processes are greatly impaired in plants, animals and humans when deprived of sunlight for a prolonged period of time. Would anybody attempt to grow roses in the darkness? If a plant is deprived of sunlight it grows colourless and sickly or even dies. If sunrays are obstructed or limited in any way the plant will bend and grow towards them in order to get hold of the light. What boxes and other coverings do to plants, clothes and apartments do to humans. Occupancy of shaded dwellings in large cities is detrimental for the health and vitality - people grow pale and anaemic, and fall suspect to many diseases. On the other hand, abundant exposure to sunlight leads to increasing of the bodily activity, cheer, humour, happiness and bolstering of the mental powers.

Abundant sunshine is of fundamental importance in treating fever, rheumatism, rickets, cancer, skin eruptions, muscular weakness breathing and digestive disorders and many other troublesome conditions. It is also the most potent chemical agent in nature which determines chemical state of our bodies by decomposing and re-combining of its numerous chemical compounds.

Sunlight is an indispensable factor of proper bodily development, function and continued active life. It dominates the chemistry of the blood, increases the number of red-blood corpuscles and haemoglobin in the blood, improves the circulation of blood and its oxygen carrying capacity. It also stimulates the growth of healthy hair, stronger and healthier bones, amplifies suppleness and tone of our skin and its resistance to infection, bolsters muscular growth and strength even without exercise (sunlight is the best masseur), speeds up elimination of toxins, aids normal nutrition and tissue repair, etc.

Sun-ripened plants are far superior in their nutritional value to those raised in obscure conditions. Even milk from animals raised in the sun contains far more vitamins and minerals. Experiments as well as experience have shown that if you give a human being an abundance of sunlight he or she will thrive on almost any kind of a diet, and if you deprive him or her of the sunlight no diet will be good enough. It is now widely perceived by the scientific establishment that sunshine is one of the most important elements of the proper nourishment. For instance: providing that we get exposed to sunshine for about fifteen minutes a few times a week, our bodies will manufacture all of the vitamin D they require.

Living organisms grow bigger, stronger and healthier under direct sun exposure. We humans tend to spend far too much time indoors where beneficial ultra-violet sunrays cannot get through the ordinary glass windows. Quartz glass windows, like those in London zoo, should be more widely used as they permit the ultra-violet rays of the sun to pass through and reach and bathe us. Inhabitants of sunlight-deprived dwellings are far more prone to distorted states of the blood, anaemia, leukaemia, weak calcium and phosphorus metabolism, rickets of both body and mind, infant mortality, etc.

Nursing mothers would be greatly benefited by sunlight as it would enable them to supply more and better quality milk to their babies and without any dependency on the cow's milk. Comparatively painless childbirth would become the norm rather than exception as it is now. Hence, all pregnant mothers should spend plenty of time outdoors whenever the sun shines, not only for their benefit but for the sake of their offspring too.

Mental capacity and alertness are greatly enhanced even by feeble sunlight. It is well known that on dark cloudy days people are more irritable, worried and lethargic and that on sunny days good cheer and happiness return.

It is very important to make a clear distinction between sunlight and sun heat. The light is beneficial to living organisms, but strong heat is not as it causes enervation and depression. Notice how birds and other animals retreat to the shade as the heat approaches.

Hiding your eyes and head behind sunglasses and hats is ridiculous. It causes the pupils of our eyes to become chronically dilated so as to take in as much of available light as possible. When the eyes are in such condition for a prolonged period of time, their exposure to sunlight becomes painful and muscles around the eyes tend to tighten and freeze in a squint in order to "protect" the eyes from "excess" light. Therefore, sunglasses are as beneficial to the eyes as crutches are beneficial to a person with weak leg muscles. Those optical crutches serve only to further weaken our eyes and their ability to cope with light. Mother Nature has created our heads and eyes adapted to sunlight which is very beneficial to them. Sunlight brings a healthy glow and enhances the beauty of our bodies. Without sunlight our eyes, heads and entire bodies weaken and become diseased.

In summary, sunlight is a profound agent of life – very important source of energy and crucial contributing factor to our health and vitality.

Another crucial factor is...

Chapter Four

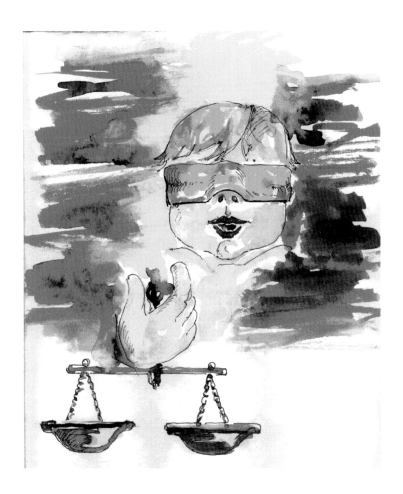

Air and Breathing

*"When the breath wanders,
the mind is unsteady,
but when the breath is still,
so is the mind still."*

(Hatha Yoga Pradipika)

AIR AND BREATHING

"When the breath wanders, the mind is unsteady, but when the breath is still, so is the mind still."
(Hatha Yoga Pradipika)

Fresh air is the essential source of vital energy. We distil the energy of the Sun through the air. We interchange telepathic messages to one another through the air. Crucially, life force enters the body with the first inhalation of air at birth. At death it departs with the last exhalation.

Importances of breathing to our bodies are manyfold. One can live only a few minutes without air and yet many people take breathing for granted. Its two basic functions are the energising of our bodies by collecting, circulating and storing vital energy through inhalation, and cleansing of toxins from the bloodstream through exhalation. Proper breathing helps maintain our body's bioelectric balance and the lack of it causes various maladies.

Every day we breathe in around 10,000 litres of air. Breathing helps to clean our lymphatic system, which is in fact our sewage system. While our heart pumps blood around, there is no pump for the lymph. It moves aided by the movement of our muscles, especially our diaphragm. Deep diaphragmatic breathing causes lymph movement some 10-15 times better than "normal" chest breathing. Diaphragmatic breathing thus aids our immune system and gives us plenty of oxygen. When our cells get enough oxygen they produce energy and function as Mother Nature intended it. And when our cells function then the whole organism functions with a sense of peace and harmony. Shallow breathing on the other hand leads to dizziness, chest pain, numbness in hands and legs, muscular spasms, neurosis etc. Some people breathe only enough to survive and as a result their bodies do not function well. The less you breathe the less healthy and vital you are. So, in order to get maximum benefit from our daily air intake, we need to learn how to breathe properly.

The essential energising element in air is the negative ion. Air gets electrically charged by sunlight. Basically, the negative ions are oxygen ions while the positive ones are carbon dioxide ions. A proper balance between the negatively and positively charged ions is very important. Negatively charged ions bring about a feeling of exhilaration and vitality. The energising vitality of negative ions in air is being destroyed by pollutants such as dust, smoke and toxic chemicals, all of which are charged by positive ions that neutralise the negative ones and thus rob air of its vitality. That is why spending as much time as possible in an open and pollution-free environment is of the paramount importance.

The human brain is one of the most energy hungry organs of our body. In order to work optimally it needs to be bathed in a constant supply of oxygen-enriched blood. If there is a shortage of oxygen, the nerve cells undergo profound destructive changes and hardly ever recover. And, although the plentiful supply of oxygen is in the surrounding air – circa 21% of the air about us – for one reason or another we seldom take in enough of it.

One also must bear in mind the fact that the vital negative ion energy from air is being assimilated by the tissues located in our nostrils and sinuses and thus the inhalation should always be through the nose. Our nostrils filter, warm and moisten incoming air making it much cleaner and friendlier to the lungs than air taken through the mouth.

Equally important is to breathe primarily with our diaphragm rather than become circumstantial tensed shallow chest breathers. That way, the diaphragm contracts and stomach protrudes allowing our lungs to expand and get filled with air. Diaphragmatic breathing greatly enhances blood circulation, promotes the production of haemoglobin in the bone marrow, increases respiratory efficiency and overall lung capacity, helps the process of elimination, boosts natural immunity to illness and thus conserves vital energy.

Scientific research has revealed that most of you access less than 20% of your breathing capacity. That leaves you short of energy and compromises your health and vitality. What's more, starting with the onset of adulthood, your respiratory capacity declines at the rate of 1-3% for every year of your life. So, unless you do something in order to improve or at least maintain it, your respiratory capacity will deteriorate and with it your well-being will deteriorate too.

For the reasons mentioned above, breathing exercises should become an integral part of your daily routine. Conscious attention to your breathing will calm, energise and integrate your body, your mind and your soul. The benefits of practising it are beyond measure and will last for as long as you continue to practise.

Here is my favourite one: Find a tranquil place and lay down on your back with your legs bent. Inhale and try to take in as much air as you can while raising your stomach muscles and keeping your rib cage relaxed. Hold your breath for as long as you comfortably can. Now exhale and using only abdominal muscles push all of the air out of your lungs. Exhalation should last twice as long as inhalation. Doing this will make you feel as if there is an invigorating energy source flowing into you. Repeat this process ten times. The most beneficial times to do the exercise are early in the morning, or around midnight, or after the rain. At those times air is rich in ozone which is highly important for your health and vitality.

Skin breathing and its profound significance for our health and our vitality have to be mentioned here, too. The outer surface of skin has many tiny openings known as pores. Air penetrates the pores and brings vital energy into the body. This energy is immediately taken up and utilised by the blood. Moreover, via the air and through the pores of the skin, telepathic messages reach our nervous system. Pores also discharge poisonous gases and fumes via the process of perspiration. If they happen to get clogged with any kind of waste substance, or cosmetic powder for that matter, pores are unable to perform their functions and as a consequence the organism suffers. Hence, the cleanliness of the skin is a prerequisite for both its breathing and poison elimination.

Breathing, both through lungs and skin, is highly important for the subsistence of our mental faculties. Our emotional states are also greatly affected by the way we breathe. Besides, remember: the freer your spirit is, the freer your breathing is. Many nervous disorders have their roots in insufficient breathing and in poor air quality.

Clean air is the best tonic for the body, mind and soul, while impure air is a catalyst of weakness and disease. Make sure your home and your workplace are well ventilated at all times.

In the next chapter we will contemplate upon...

Chapter Five

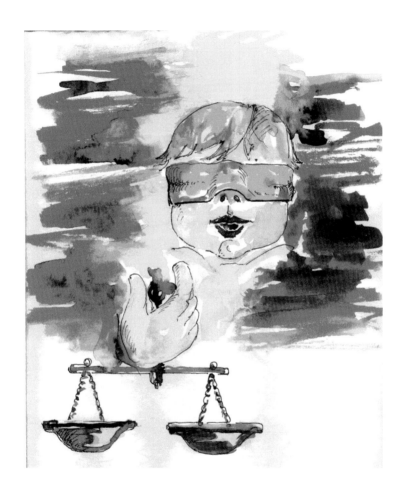

Water and Hydration

*"Water, in moderation,
cannot hurt anybody."*

(Mark Twain)

WATER AND HYDRATION

"Water, in moderation, cannot hurt anybody."
(Mark Twain)

Now, after you have laughed at the above wanton understatement, please take a moment to think earnestly about the significance of water for your well-being.

Around 70% of our planet is covered by water and circa 70% of our bodies is water. Our brains and our blood are in excess of 80% water content. Water is the main ingredient of all living matter. Owing to its high content of vital energy, water is necessary for almost all bodily functions, and almost everything dissolves in water. Above all, water gives form to cells and actively participates in their reactions. Hence, every structure of the body needs to receive its, by nature predetermined, share of water and nutrients transported with it, or body functioning will become impaired.

Human beings can survive even if they lose 50% of sugar, fat and protein. Loss of 10% of water from your body is harmful and loss of 20% of water can be fatal. Your organism does not have a reservoir for storing water, so any quantity lost has to be replaced by prompt water consumption. The constancy of water in our body not only provides nourishment to cells and brings away from them the refuse for elimination, but is also the very prerequisite for existence of life. The founder of physiology, Claude Bernard, referred to the phenomenon of life as *"the totality of the circulating fluids of the organism"*.

We humans are considered to be air-inhabiting creatures however, as our cells and all living elements of our body are in contact with fluid, we are water inhabitants as well. Therefore, it is crystal clear that our diet should contain at least 70% of food rich in water. That ensures proper functioning and cleansing of our bodily system. Otherwise, our system gets clogged. How are you doing here?

You may have heard the dogmatic advice to drink at least eight glasses of water between meals every day. Others say: drink water only when thirsty. Who is right? Whom should we believe? Who shall we follow? Well, I do not know. I have practised both and now tend to believe that one should listen to what the body calls for. The wisdom of the body takes into the consideration the climate you live in, the season of the year, type of work you do, food you eat etc. For example, if one eats plenty of water rich fruits and vegetables the body will call for lot less water. On the other hand, eating of spicy, greasy and concentrated foods creates an irritation of digestive tract, which is commonly mistaken for thirst. Drinking water in such instances will not satisfy the "thirst" at all and will only serve to dilute the digestive juices, carry them away and cause indigestion. And, while water cannot satisfy this "thirst", the digestive juices can and will do so. Give them a chance and your irresistible desire for water will pass away.

Your sensation of thirst, if unobstructed by any of your desires and habits that are at odds with natural order, will adjust to the above-mentioned factors and hence it will regulate the stability of water in the body. Listen to your body, please.

Insufficient water intake causes constipation, loss of muscle tone and reduction in muscle performance, makes your skin get dry, itchy and saggy, troubles the regulation and maintenance of body temperature, impairs proper kidney functioning and toxin elimination, slows burning up of fats stored in your body, curtails your mental capacity, etc.

Excessive water drinking, on the other hand, lowers the ability of the blood to carry oxygen, causes one to sweat more and generally weakens the body. If sustained over prolonged period of time, this habit can cause low sodium levels in your blood – a condition which in itself is life threatening.

Carbonated beverages, caffeine and alcohol cannot be used as a substitute for drinking water. On the contrary, they cause your body to lose water through increased urination and actually increase your bodily water requirements. A habitual preference for the taste of these beverages reduces the urge to drink water when they are not available and leads to dehydration.

You may be surprised to hear that your body loses water even while you sleep. Therefore it is advisable to start your day with a glass of water rather than a cup of coffee and thus get your body's metabolic reactions going unimpaired from the outset. And here is something else that you ought to pay attention to: the more yellow your urine is, the more water you should take in. It is an unmistakable indicator of the level of your body's immediate water requirement.

Without water a seed cannot grow and produce a new plant. Without adequate water consumption your body cannot work effectively. Such is the importance of water for the miracle of life. Yet, in excess of any sort, water can be harmful. Democritus summed it up nicely by saying: *"Water can be both good and bad, useful and dangerous. To the danger, however, a remedy has been found: learning to swim."* Learn to "swim" through your life by listening to your body and living in harmony with Nature.

Now let's examine the another important factor of health and vitality...

Chapter Six

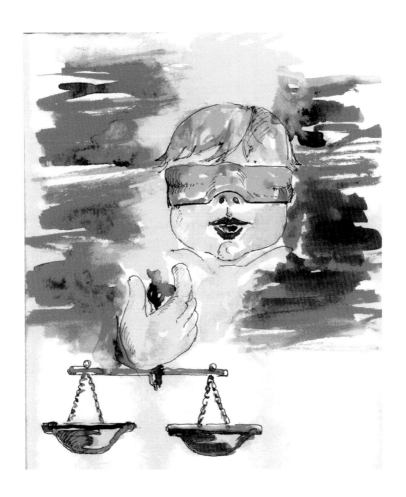

Nutrition Mission

*"Subdue your appetites, my dears,
and you've conquered human nature."*

(Charles Dickens)

NUTRITION MISSION

"Subdue your appetites, my dears, and you've conquered human nature." (Charles Dickens)

Several years ago, my eating practices were the first area of my search for possible reasons and answers to my arthritic condition. Having read about the adverse influences of excess uric acid and animal protein on our well-being, I decided to stop consuming animal products for a period of a few weeks. The improvement that followed was phenomenal, so I have never considered going back to the old ways of eating. That change was the starting point of my recovery and my health transformation.

Our bodies are composed of tens of trillions of cells. In order for our bodies to be healthy and vital those cells must be functional and healthy first. To meet that requirement they need fuel. The fuel from which our cells derive energy and help our bodies to function well are the vital nutrients that come from the food we eat.

A great number of people take in what their self-gratifying mind asks for instead of consuming food that meets the necessary requirements of their bodies. Self-indulgence soon turns into addiction. Burdened with the weight of food taken in to feed those greedy desires of their minds, their bodies suffer and their brains struggle to govern their thoughts.

According to scientists, the human dental structure and digestive system are both designed to process fibrous food. Yet, tendencies are more towards very restrictive diets which are, due to their narrowness, rather damaging.

By making small changes in your dietary habits you can provide your body with more than enough energy for it to complete all its daily routines. Discipline over appetites and passions is the master key.

Although many books on diet and nutrition have been written, it is hard to find two authors who agree on particular issues. So, to whom should you listen? To your body, in harmony with the laws of Nature, of course. Your body will tell you everything, if only you will pay attention. Below are mentioned some general guidelines in order to help you draw your own conclusions.

Generally, your diet should meet your body's requirements and they are: an adequate amount of protein (amino acids) for building and repair of your bodily tissues; a sufficient amount of adequate sugars, vitamins and minerals for normal daily functions of the body; enough fats and carbohydrates for supply of heat and energy to your body. All of these food elements are present in abundance in fresh fruit, fresh vegetables, grains and nuts.

Food combining is vital for proper digestion, obtaining maximum nutrition and energy. We consume staggering amount of approximately 500 kg of food every year. Different food types require different digestive juices for their digestion. When very different foods are eaten together, different digestive juices get in action and their chemical reactions often obstruct one another prolonging digestion and robbing you of energy. For that reason, proteins and carbo-hydrates should not be eaten at the same time. Fats also slow down the digestion of proteins and if you have to have them together then have a salad as well in order to minimise those negative effects.

The main source of fats, cholesterol above all, is meat. Excess fat causes heart troubles and the clogging of your blood vessels. Coagulated red blood cells cannot get through capillaries, oxygen distribution gets obstructed and, as a result, your cells weaken and then mutate or die. And those blockages can be fatal indeed.

Meat is also considered by many to be the main source of protein. The underlying fad of many diet regimes is that we need plenty of protein for energy. There is a big craze amongst young generations, especially those "body building" ones. Led by some diet regimes they tend to eat food that is 50-70% protein, which is totally unnecessary. There is a loose scientific consensus that one gram of protein per one kilogram of your body weight a day is more than enough. When do you need protein most? When you are a baby, of course. What percentage of human mother's milk is protein? Only around 1.5%, as there is in most fruit. Excess protein creates excess nitrogen in your body and that leads to fatigue. Those guys with bulky muscles cannot endure long runs – they get tired easily and quickly. And we are supposed to be the endurance creatures.

Some people think that if they do not eat meat their bones might weaken. Meat contains a lot of uric acid which drains calcium from your body. In order to get rid of acid your organism draws calcium from reserves, and when there are no reserves then the necessary calcium gets drawn from the bones and teeth. The more meat you eat the weaker your bones will be. The strongest bones are in herbivores such as the elephant and gorilla. Furthermore, uric acid from excess meat consumption poisons your bloodstream, irritates your tendons and joints and causes arthritis.

If you have to eat meat, eat it sensibly: maximum at one meal a day; combine it properly with other food (eg: salad is okay, potatoes are not); let the source be kosher (drained from uric acid). And chew this: Carnivores in Nature eat meat raw so that none of its nutritional elements are lost in the way they are lost in the process of cooking.

Milk and dairy products promote creation of mucus and fat in your body and clog your system. Circa 20% of population do not secrete enough lactacin, enzyme required for digestion of sugar from milk. Many allergies happen as a result. While it is adequate in the earliest period of life providing it comes from own species, milk is inadequate food in adulthood due to the excess of alkalies. In experiments, rabbits fed on cow's milk died of acidosis. According to statistical data, the mortality rate of babies bottle-fed during their first year of life is seven times greater than of the breast-fed ones. Cows do not drink cow's milk, why would you or your baby? The breast-fed infants get a better start in life, grow and develop more naturally and have greater resistance to illness. And, let me emphasise one more fact: pasteurisation of milk alters the calcium salts in it to the extent that they are no longer of any use to the consumer.

Fruit is the most perfect food. It is highly nutritious, contains plenty of water, takes very little of your energy and time for its digestion and with its fibre content also helps in the cleansing of your organism. It strengthens your capillaries, prevents clothing of blood, reduces risk of internal bleeding and helps the functioning of your heart. The old catchphrase: "An apple a day keeps the doctor away," sums it up nicely. And keep this in mind: Fruit should not be taken together or after other food. It should be eaten alone and on an empty stomach.

Try and eat only when hungry and not to please your craving for food. Do not eat during or straight after strenuous physical or mental effort. Refrain from overloading your stomach right before going to sleep. Otherwise, your stomach will have to work hard while you are trying to rest. You should also refrain from eating when in any sort of pain or when under stress. Chew all food properly, as this practice will greatly help the process of digestion. Whenever possible, eat organically grown food as it is free of herbicides and pesticides. You should not drink water during or right after the meal as it dilutes the digestive juices and slows down the process of digestion.

You should also remember that for proper and complete nutrition, apart from consumption of proper foods in proper combinations, your body has to be able to digest that food, assimilate the nutrients and eliminate the waste. If any of these constituents is impaired the process of nutrition is affected and as a result all your bodily functions and processes suffer. Factors which can affect the process of nutrition are your mental states, love practices, exercise regime, work and play mode, the quality of your sleep and rest (relaxation), the amount of oxygen and sunshine your body gets etc. Whatever the negative influence is, it must be corrected so that your body can properly utilise the food and get the full benefit from it.

Moderation is of no value if you eat white bread, refined oil, fried food, pasteurised food, denatured cereals, refined salt, puddings, coffee, refined sugar, etc. as they are loaded with calories and low in all important cellular nutrients.

Common addictive substances such as sugar, caffeine and alcohol greatly undercut your health and vitality and in turn diminish your ability to fully enjoy your life. Furthermore, all addictions undermine your self-honesty, as their illusionary values require dishonest realisations, and as a result lower your self-esteem, competence and prosperity. People who consume these substances may well think they are enjoying life, when in fact they are drug addicts. The feelings and actions of the addicts get deceived, the initial acute poisoning of the digestive system, the nervous system, the blood, and the organs of the body becomes chronic, and when the consequences arise they go to the doctor to cure the effects of their "enjoyment". Finally, they kill themselves with the prescription drugs while "curing" themselves of those consequences. How foolish. So much for the modern educational system that does not educate, but produces generations of individuals whose spirits are being amputated in the process instead.

The damaging effects of such addictive substances do not usually arise after a single occurrence, but are rather cumulative. The real and lasting harmful effects of the addictions are equal to their apparent and temporary beneficial effects. Seemingly they make our bodies feel stronger, while in fact they weaken us. As there are not immediate symptoms of poisoning, many people tend to even deny harmful character of the addictive substances they habitually use. The truth is that any initial false sense of satisfaction, or of seemingly increased vigour and enjoyment, which these substances cause, is followed by the harmful effects and depression. The reason for this is the expenditure of vital energy that caused the exhilaration in the first place. The stimulation that the addictive substances bring about is the excitement of irritation and not the invigoration and revitalisation of nutrition.

The most destructive of them all is refined sugar. This sedative causes more metabolic and psychological harm than all other addictive substances combined. When sugar cane or sugar beets are processed, the bulk, fibre, vitamins and minerals are being removed from them and this simple carbohydrate – refined sugar is produced. As such, it causes our bodies to draw these missing elements from the reserves, in order to utilise it. Sugar arouses and increases action, but at the same time decreases the power of action and functioning of the stimulated organs. Your body stores sugar as fat layers primarily around your waist, thighs and chest. The next in line of attack are your major internal organs, heart and kidneys. Hyperactivity, obesity, ageing, diabetes, tooth decay, cataracts, heart disease, cancer and other degenerative disorders are to a great extent the effects of refined sugar consumption. In spite of all this, sugar is liberally being added into many processed foods and promoted as a natural energy source. A friend of mine was able to stop taking many of the drugs prescribed to him and feels much better than he did for a long time, by simply eliminating sugar from his diet.

Stimulant caffeine consumed with coffee, chocolate and cola beverages affects functioning of your kidneys and pancreas. If excessive and sustained over a prolonged period of time, this habit not only causes depression, loss of sleep, spasm of muscles, but is also considered to be life threatening as it stimulates your organism to borrow the energy from tomorrow's reserves for today's use. That may relax you for the moment, but one-day it eventually catches up with you. On the other hand, experiments have shown that tumour-like nodules in breasts disappeared in more than half of the women observed once they stopped consuming coffee, tea, cola drinks and chocolate.

I have heard: During the cocoa harvesting and processing season its aroma attracts swarms of a certain insect. As they wander around the plantations, these insects get harvested together with the cocoa, piled in heaps, placed in bins, and then processed. Consequently they end up as a "condiment" to your favourite chocolate, cookies, cakes, etc. Wonder what that insect is? It is a cockroach... Bon appétit!

Alcohol addiction irritates and impairs every organ of the body. It coagulates (or cooks) the protoplasm of the cells of the body, causes a sludging of red blood cells and the clogging of blood capillaries that leads to oxygen-starvation and dehydration of brain cells and ultimately to a death of those brain cells. As the brain cell replication is considered to be between extremely slow to non-existent, the effects of alcoholism are permanently damaging. It is well known that alcohol is not a stimulant, but a narcotic that dulls your senses, awareness, intelligence and reasoning. The functioning powers of the nervous system, liver, heart, lungs, kidneys, muscles, arteries and every other vital organ are gradually destroyed by alcohol. Alcohol does not actually give any strength to the user, even though the user may "feel" such an effect. It rather wastes strength. Vital energy does not go out of alcohol into the user's body. In fact, alcohol causes the vital energy to be exhausted from the body, as the body attempts to expel it. Even when taken in small quantities alcohol lowers your body's resistance to diseases.

The more addicted you are to the apparent effects – the more you crave, and the less satisfied and the more unhappy you are. By quickly breaking those detrimental habits you measurably improve the quality of your life. That requires self-awareness first, then self-honesty, and finally commitment. Please bear in mind that all the effort will be in vain unless the purity of heart is attained through a spiritual fast. The best way to get rid of those habits is to challenge your false beliefs, see the things as they truly are, make an unwavering decision to change, and then follow it through irrevocably, wholeheartedly, and forever. And as soon as you change your perceptions your habits will begin to change, and your old beliefs will stop bothering you and disappear. So, go on - do it! Since you have stayed with me thus far I know you will.

One caveat: Synthetic supplements do not work. Some of you may have tried to compensate for your inadequate dietary habits by taking synthetic vitamins and minerals. The evidence against it is overwhelming. Let me mention here some findings of the research on administering the vitamin supplements: A group of rabbits given synthetic vitamin C did not show any increase of ascorbic acid in their blood while in a group given raw cabbage, levels of ascorbic acid did ascend significantly. Similarly, chicken fed with natural vitamin

D extract from cod-liver oil grew stronger and lived longer than those given synthetic vitamin D of whom 60% died before reaching maturity. The message is clear, make sure you consume plenty of live food and if you do need any supplements take ones derived from live sources.

Between 65 and 70% of the western-world population are overweight by their own estimation. Those people, not satisfied with the normal demands of their bodies for food, tend to resort to various food condiments, relishes and dressings in order to stimulate their appetite so as to be able to eat more. People who habitually eat for pleasure beyond their digestive capacity and who pay no attention to their actual food requirements do overwork their entire organisms, poison their bodies and wreck their health and vitality. It is believed that overeating, which is also referred to as food-addiction, kills more people than famine.

Face it – you become fat because you are hoarding inside your body in order to appease your miserly mind, deep-seated in blind and lustful ignorance. You keep putting in your mouth and in your stomach many things that you should be putting in your heart. It is a crime against your body to eat when you are not hungry. If you really desire sound health and vitality, eat only when you are truly hungry and do not consume more food than your body truly needs.

Fasting, on the other hand, can be very beneficial for the health. It is an old practice, referred to even in the Bible, known to help eliminate toxins from body, increase energy levels and speed-up recovery from illness. Even so, the medical profession still favours prescribing drugs. By the way, an animal fasts when ill – why wouldn't you?

In order to tease your mind, let me mention here some notably distinguished vegetarians: Socrates, Pithagoras,

Lao Tzu, Confucius, The Buddha, Christ, Da Vinci, Seneca, Voltaire, Newton, Tolstoy, Twain, Van Gogh, Tesla ... Not a bad group of people to look up to. This is not to say that you should become a vegetarian. It is only an option. You are the only person who should make the choice for yourself.

A panacea has not been found, and probably never will be found. It is up to us all to search and find the best ways and means for preserving our physiological stability, or at least stop jeopardising it. Nature has given us the autonomic system for self-regulation of physiological processes. It is our mind illusions born out of unawareness and our lack of discipline that disturb that harmony.

Good nutrition can make a great difference to the functioning of our bodies. Consumption of wholesome foods rather than denatured and adulterated products is the key and the foundation of your health and vitality. This fact has been known for a long time, and yet, a very few of us make practical application of this knowledge. Instead, led by some "higher authority" in the form of other people or through advertising, the majority of people remain in pursuit of phoney pleasures, indulge themselves in bad dietary habits and inevitably become enslaved by them. To accept authority for truth instead of accepting truth for authority is foolish. To believe that your bad habits are actually the "good things in life" and that by breaking them nothing would be gained is insane. Are you aware of the fact that no other living creature on this planet but man would eat excessively or eat anything that is harmful to its body? Are you aware of the tricks and games of your mind? Free your body from the tyranny and manipulations of your twisted self-indulgent mind, please, and eat according to your inner need guided by awareness of your non-attached soul. Fulfil your bodily needs and drop your cravings, your attachment to desires – attachments that get in the way of your body's wisdom, attachments that eat you. Truly, that will add years to your life and also life to your years. The law of Nature has it that sooner or later the ignorant ones will perish. To obey the law of Nature is neither restriction nor self-sacrifice but our path to and prerequisite for sound health and vitality.

Eat wisely guided by truth.

Chapter Seven

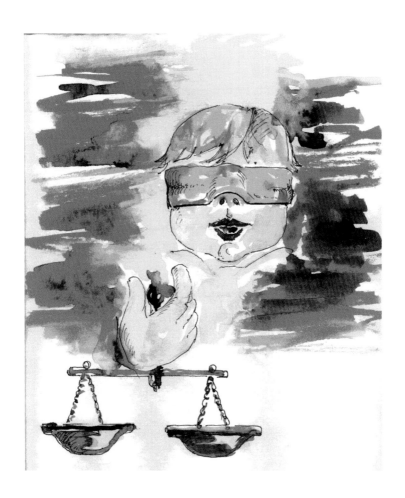

Motion and Exercise

"The human body,
is the best picture of the human soul."

(Ludwig Wittgenstein)

MOTION AND EXERCISE

"The human body, is the best picture of the human soul."
(Ludwig Wittgenstein)

When my stomach collapsed and the flesh started disappearing from my body, I thought I'd better refrain from exercising in order to preserve the energy. This idea may have been a sound one as a temporary measure, but as I followed it – it became a habit. As the time went by and as my condition steadied, I still remained pretty passive physically. Why? I do not know. I just did. You can imagine how much "good" that did to me. My body was getting weaker and weaker and with it my peace of mind. One day I took a good look of myself in the mirror, saw the grievous picture for what it truly was, and remembered my mother's wise words, spoken to me when I was a teenager, which implied that freedom from pains and strains in life is best attained by living a life of acute alertness and motion. Awareness is marvellous medicine which liberates vital energy and unifies the body, the mind and the soul. It arouse my constrained will and set it free. My spirit became indestructible. The rest is history.

Your body is designed to move. Movement is life; life is energy. Energy in movement is delightful, however when stagnant it turns sour, it turns bitter, it turns burdensome. Movement boosts up your endorphin levels and thus increases your strength, stamina, suppleness, or – in one word – energy. So, get up and get moving, stretch, lift and throw things. Exercise is good for you and so is making love or dancing. Find out what suits you best and do it. The more active you are, the healthier and more vital you are. Your body can be either a source of pleasure or a source of pain. You clearly have the choice.

Exercise is certainly one of the most important vital tonics for the body. It invariably conveys vigour and activity of all the organs, sustains the symmetrical development of the body and secures and maintains the integrity of all bodily functions. Through exercise the whole body gets strengthened and invigorated. The lack of exercise weakens the body and diminishes its physiological powers. This is truly an irrevocable law of life.

Adopting sensible lifestyle habits is of paramount importance. Our ancestors were hunters and gatherers who had to constantly be in motion in order to survive and live. With the arrival of technology modern man has adopted a sedentary lifestyle and he is suffering because of that. Even manual workers suffer due to specialism and one-sided repetitive tendencies of their jobs. Survival of contemporary man no longer depends on motion. Throughout the day we sit in the office, sit in the vehicle, or sit on the sofa and watch television. Motion is no longer part of our daily routine. Our bodies, starved of the movement necessary for its functioning and maintenance, communicate to us about this deficiency through the language of pain. The ultimate lack of motion is death, right? Do you really want to go down that road sooner than you need to?

Through motion and exercise we create a strong aerobic base and also keep our bodily biochemistry balanced. Our bodies get more oxygen, more energy and more strength. Bodily endurance, proper posture, agility and co-ordination are developed. The quality of the bones, the flexibility of the joints, the strength of the heart and blood vessels, the powers of digestion and assimilation, the efficiency of elimination, circulation of blood and lymph, lung capacity and respiration, the tone of muscles and virtually every tissue are all dependant on exercise. Physical exercise trains the mind and develops our vital organs. As long as the balance is maintained, it doesn't matter how you exercise.

The most effective way of generating more energy through movement is aerobic exercise. Aerobic means "with oxygen" as that kind of exercise burns oxygen without creating deficit, hence can be done over longer period of time. As a result, your lungs process more air with less effort and your heart gets stronger and pumps more blood with fewer beats. Blood inflow to your muscles gets better and in general the quantity of blood in your body increases. In short, you expand the capacity of your body to absorb the oxygen, blend it with essential nutrients and create energy. With that you greatly improve your endurance and regulate your metabolism.

There are several formulas for calculating your optimum aerobic heart rate. One that has worked for me best is: 170 minus your age. Also, a pretty good indicator that you are training within your aerobic zone is if you can talk effortlessly while you exercise.

The duration of your exercising regime depends on oxygen intake. The shorter it is the more vigorous exercise should be in order to achieve steady heart rhythm with optimum number of beats. If exercise is less vigorous and if your body requires more oxygen to steady the heart rate, then you need to prolong its duration. Your aim is to exercise over longer periods of time while totally enjoying yourself, free from muscle cramps, shortness of breath and tiredness.

Anaerobic exercise builds your muscles; aerobic exercise builds your well-being. Proper exercising regime will propel you to towering health and versatile vitality. And if you maintain it for one year without any breaks, you will create a "habit" for life. What a "habit" to have!

As well as being significant for the maintenance of health and vitality, physical exercise is a very valuable and effective means for restoring health. Many bodily deformities and abnormalities such as spinal curvature, stiff neck, round shoulders, bow legs, flat foot, shortened muscles and ligaments, fallen stomach and womb, etc. can be corrected via specially designed exercises. For optimum results, these corrective exercises are best performed under the supervision of an expert.

More than a half of the population of the industrialised world are not sufficiently physically active and around a quarter of that population are "couch potatoes" – not active at all. Absence of physical activity is responsible for the sudden downfall of many famous and successful people right at their peak (Harold Wilson, Elvis Presley, and others) as well as of a great many common people. Firm, symmetrical, beautiful bodies were worshiped by ancient civilisations. Wild animals are strong and well proportioned as they move a lot driven by the urge of hunger and survival. On the other hand, domestic animals have their food given to them, do not exercise their bodies and as a result they become fat and lazy. Such routines inevitably lead to shortening of life span and to premature deaths.

Modern man has put the importance of intellect development to the fullest extent, but at the expense of movement and physical exercise. This lack of movement is very dangerous since motion is essential to energy and blood circulation. As a consequence, the body becomes soft, flabby, out of symmetry and out of shape. He has forgotten the fact that his intellect cannot give its best unless his body is able to function properly, and he suffers for that. It is high time for a change in the physical activity habits of population and what a better place to start the process than at our educational institutions.

Motion and exercise are energy consuming while rest and sleep are energy replenishing states. Both are required for sustenance of life and maintenance of health and vitality. They should be carefully cultivated as our mental, emotional and spiritual powers are inseparably linked to them. Powerful intellect must be backed by a vigorous body. Nature has put them together in perfect concord and this balance must be maintained or both will suffer. The solution is simple: keep on moving and exercising regularly and then rest sufficiently so that your body can recuperate for the new challenges. Keeping this equation balanced is absolutely essential prerequisite for preserving your health and vitality. Otherwise, the imbalance may lead to burn-out, ill-health, injury, or in one word – pain.

One of the skills of movement therapy, which profoundly complements all other exercise practices and enhances their effectiveness, is the art of massage. Massage is an excellent medium for increasing the range of movement and, like any other exercise, improves blood circulation, encourages lymphatic flow, relaxes and tones muscles, stretches the connective tissue of joints, balances the body temperature, releases trapped emotions and bodily tensions, relieves stress and anxiety, enhances breathing, clears blockages from the energy channels and aids digestion. It also helps you rejuvenate your sense organs and your inner organs through employment of your vital energy, improve your posture and facial expression, integrate your body through touch and heightened awareness, and generally – create feelings of harmony, relaxation, joy and freedom.

Yoga is another exercise discipline that is in part physical although generally holistic and definitely one of the most complex. The physical domain of Yoga contains a series of exercises and specific postures, which greatly help you to attain control over your body, its organs, muscles and glands, as well as help you greatly improve your posture and the circulation of blood and vital energy. In order for this physical aspect of Yoga to be effective it must be complemented with breathing and mental concentration exercises. That will make you more sensitive, more open, more alive. Unquestionably, it is the significant way for attainment of a self-mastery of your body, mind and spirit – the whole of you. Yoga is a profound tool for integration, growth and achievement of magnificent health and vitality.

Mother Nature's great antidote for pain is a simple exercise called laughter. Laughter is a magical catalyst for health. It is rest to the tired and sunshine to the sad and discouraged. It creates much happiness and induces health. When we laugh, our blood vessels expand, the blood flow increases and our circulatory system functions more effectively, bolstering our overall sense of well-being. Laughter, or even a genuine smile, transmits a nectar-like secretion in a form of loving energy – energy that heals. So, do not ever forget what it is to laugh and feel good laughing.

Lovemaking (or sex, if you will) is one of the primary existential manifestations of motion which is indispensable to our health and vitality. It is a shared experience, shared self-expression – the most energetic physical, emotional and spiritual union in surrender, and communication of love between lovers, absorbed in the moment, wholly present, free of repressive feelings (such as guilt and inhibition) and expectations (of results) rooted in society's misguided conditioning. Without its spiritual dimension – tied to the mere energy release, in mere pursuit of pleasure, for mere indulgence – lovemaking is mechanical and leads to a compulsive repetition, emptiness, feeling less than human, neurosis, frustration, and ultimately to pain. Blended with the power of spirit, it becomes an inexhaustible source of natural, spontaneous, vibrant energy that transmits in waves, ebbing and flowing, throughout our intertwined trembling bodies, throughout our melting hearts, throughout our merging souls, and in its cosmic dance creates undreamed levels of ecstasy. *"My soul glowed from the fire of your fire; your world was a whispering water, at the river of my heart"*, wrote ancient Persian poet Rumi. Such intimate blending of flesh and spirit, such transcendent communion, such disappearance of our beings in the clouds of utter ecstasy, bring joy from fulfilment and relaxation that greatly enhance our well-being.

Physical activity not only increases circulation and muscle elasticity but it also refreshes the brain, causing it to increasingly produce the chemical endorphin which relieves pain, reduces stress, gives rise to a blissful feeling of mild euphoria and brings vibrancy to life.

Our physical states are greatly dependent on our feelings. And, our feelings are also greatly affected by motion. Feelings of fitness, grace, beauty, poise and a joy of living cannot be had without motion.

Commit yourself to creating greater emotional strength and radiant passion – the spring of vitality – in your life through motion.

Chapter Eight

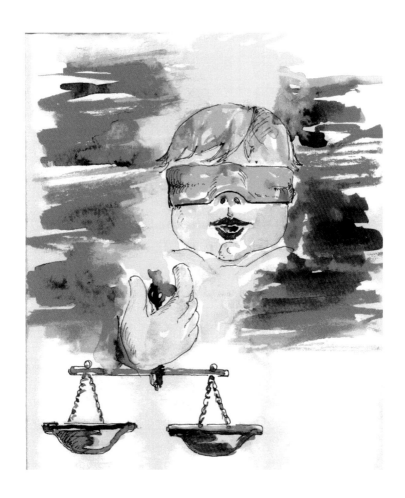

Environment and Pollution

*"Our bodies are our gardens...
our wills are gardeners."*

(William Shakespeare)

ENVIRONMENT AND POLLUTION

"Our bodies are our gardens...our wills are gardeners."
(William Shakespeare)

Nowadays humankind is reaping the rewards of the technological breakthroughs of the last two centuries that have brought an ever-increasing productivity and raising standards of living. On the other hand, the same accomplishments are also responsible for the ruthless destruction of our planet, for genocide on a massive scale and for a gradual diminishing of quality of our lives. Man has divorced science from ethics and as a consequence, the equilibrium between human beings and the environment has been broken.

With every passing day, two species disappear from the face of the Earth. Entire forests have vanished for the sake of certain vested interests of the socio-economic elite (for instance: indiscriminate production and distribution of second-rate newspapers and magazines). Rising levels of carbon-dioxide in the atmosphere and subsequent global warming in turn brings about melting of the ice-caps, floods, destruction of the environment, loss of life, etc. Likewise, the life-shielding ozone layer that surrounds our planet is being damaged with every rocket and satellite passing through it, causing hazardous rays to start entering the atmosphere and harming life on Earth. The whole ecosystems are grossly endangered and not even the humankind is being spared. And we are being advised to use sun-creams, lotions, and sunglasses for our protection. How ironical!

Do you happen to know how long you can expect to live? Statisticians have compiled the data from the lives of millions of people and given us their predictions. The omens are not rosy at all. Most of us are passionately eager to prove statisticians wrong and to live longer. How can we do that? Well, there is an answer, a conceivable way of achieving this. The following paragraphs should give you a clue.

In the laboratory experimenting at the Rockefeller Institute, living chicken cells were kept in an environment with all-necessary requirements and pollution free for a period of over thirty years. Then the experiment was abandoned with a conclusion that the cells could live indefinitely under the given circumstances. I am sure you know how long chicken's life span is. So, how about us, humans? Could we live a few hundred years? Could we live indefinitely? Of course! It is simple: do something about toxins – both those from the environment, as well as those free radicals that biochemical processes of our bodies generate. Those free radicals are in fact the particles that lack electrons. As such they are very unstable, charged with energy, and looking for anything in your body – be it your DNA or amino-acids – to join. Than they virtually steal electrons and thus trigger the process of oxidation, or "rusting", obstruct self-regulating functions of your bodies, lead to their deterioration, and speed-up ageing process. Do everything you can to avoid them or help your body to fight them with antioxidants like vitamin C. Take the example of the Chinese herbalist Lee Ching-Yuen who died in 1933 at the chronological age of 256. Biologically, he looked about 50 years old, was vigorously healthy and vital throughout his life, and married 24 times. The "secret" to his remarkably long and active life was adherence to the laws of Nature and thoughtful evasion of stress and other forms of pollution. By conquering toxemia we could achieve eternal immortality.

Our bodies react to everything in the environment. While useful substances get assimilated and used, harmful substances get eliminated or at least our bodies attempt to establish defence against them in one way or another. These defensive reactions of our bodies are directly proportional to the level of destructiveness of the harmful substances. A degree of bodily toleration defines the speed and effectiveness of the reactions against pollutants.

Common and extensive abuse of chemicals such as herbicides and pesticides have increasingly been linked to various neuro-degenerative disorders that turn the simplest movement into a battle between the brain and nerves. The recent studies at the University of Maastricht in Holland have concluded that many mental ailments found in farmers and gardeners are the direct result of their contact with afore-mentioned chemical agents.

Aerosols like deodorants and other sprays are harmful. School of Medicine at "St. George's" hospital in London has registered over one hundred deaths from inhalation of deodorants and anti-perspirants since year 1971, when the records begun.

How about other air pollutants? Aboveground nuclear explosions have released deadly substances like strontium-90 and iodine-131 into the atmosphere, their fallout contaminating the air in our living environment. These radioactive particles are well-known cancer-causing agents. Emissions from fossil fuel-burning power plants cause air pollution and climate change. Apart from carbon dioxide, other harmful substances like led, sulphur dioxide, mercury, nitrogen oxides and many others are found in the air we breathe. They also impair or even block sunshine. Sunlight is highly beneficial to the process of thinking, creativity, as well as for proper work of our hearts and lungs.

Antiquated water and sewer systems are failing too. Vast amounts of untreated sewage pours into waterways from those ageing systems designed to overflow when it rains causing serious public health concerns. Problems such as contamination of drinking water, beach closures, damage to fish and shellfish stocks, are common nowadays. Yet very little progress has been made in upgrading those systems due to a "shortage" of funds.

Tap water is in many cases a major culprit in causing a variety of disorders - a far greater number of fatalities comes as a consequence of drinking impure water. Chlorine and fluoride that are routinely added to our drinking water are both known as toxic and cancer causing agents. Claims that fluoride protects our teeth have not been either substantiated by statistical data or proven by science. What's more, those chemical substances do not remove parasites and microbes from the water. When we consume low-grade water over a prolonged period of time, we harm our bodies. Hence, we should refrain from drinking tap water unless we filter it or distil it and make it less harmful. Further action is required to re-energise the living properties in our drinking water and thus enhance our health.

Various additives and "enhancers", which are regularly being added by manufacturers to processed food and many beverages in order to "improve" their taste and "please" your taste buds, are in fact harmful pollutants. The most common additive is cheap filler – refined sugar – whose negative effects I have already mentioned in the chapter 6. Also, beware of hydrogenated fats and oils, as it takes your body days to digest them, they drain your vital energy and cause havoc of the kind heroin does. There are over a dozen other ones, and together they account for circa 90% of the harm done to your bodies. Read the labels when shopping and do your utmost to avoid them.

Inadequate clothing and overclothing also weaken your body. Many people tend to overclothe themselves in winter and thus weaken reactive powers of their skins impairing its functions of absorption and elimination.

That in turn overworks kidneys and mucous membranes of the body. Wearing dark clothing excludes the beneficial sunrays from the body and weakens the whole body as a result. Sunlight is an essential factor of good health and vitality, as it is a free air circulation about the body, so one should wear light and porous clothes of light colours.

Pollution of the mind is a serious threat to our health. Anything can be instilled in our subconscious through music, words, video images, etc. What's more, we willingly accept new technology gadgets without ever questioning their harmful effects on our bodies. High-frequency and high voltage electro-transmitters, personal computers, electric blankets, television sets, mobile telephones, microwave ovens, to name but a few, do affect our health and most of you are not even aware of the dangers they bring.

We, the users, are being the part of "experiments" in hundreds of millions. As the effects do not manifest straight away, these gadgets should carry a health warning. For example, more than 50% of radio-frequency emissions (which are a harmful noninizing type of electromagnetic radiation) from a mobile telephone are absorbed by the body of the user. That saps our vital energy, causes the increase of the temperature in the head of the user and leads to damage of brain cells, headaches, dizziness, impaired vision, ringing ears, sleep disruptions, loss of memory and impaired mental attention. Furthermore, the radiation from cell phones and cellular transponder towers (antennae) causes damage of chromosomes, altered activity of certain genes, DNA damage, heart palpitations, disturbances of the digestive system, fatigue, etc.

Or, how about the use of microwave ovens? Forensic research, its astonishing evidence and subsequent conclusions of the German, Russian, American and Swiss scientists, are extremely disturbing. They are warning and nobody is listening. Nearly every household and restaurant in the "developed" western world has one. It seems that your convenience precedes your well-being. Please, set your ignorance aside and read on: Microwave cooking denatures and decays the food by the process of radiation. Microwave radiation "heated" food is neither natural (it loses up to 90% of its nutritive value), nor healthy – it is poisonous to both your body and your nervous system. Microwave oven radiation not only decays the food rendering it poisonous, but even your body's exposure to its energy-field has adverse – often cancerous – effects on the blood, brain, eyes, heart, kidneys, reproductive organs, and digestive tract. It also causes weakening of cell membranes resulting in immune system deficiencies, destabilizes and alters hormone production, promotes forming of carcinogen free radicals and other residual by-products within your body; it sparks off the stress syndrome leading to anxiety, headache, hair loss, and even heart-attack; it impairs your memory, concentration, emotional threshold, alertness, intuition, intelligence, and so on. Oh, by the way, did you know that, because of such detrimental side-effects, the Russians outlawed the use of microwave ovens in fairly faraway 1976? This kind of information should be more readily available. Sadly it is not. Instead, we are being brainwashed.

"The viewer of television, the listener to radio, the reader of magazines, is presented with a whole complex of elements – all the way from ingenious rhetoric to carefully selected data and statistics – to make it easy for him to 'make up his own mind' with the minimum of difficulty and effort. But the packaging is often done so effectively that the viewer, listener, or reader does not make up his own mind at all. Instead he inserts a packaged opinion into his mind, somewhat like inserting a cassette into a

cassette player. He than pushes a button and 'plays back' the opinion whenever it seems appropriate to do so. He has performed acceptability without having to think," emphasised beautifully the chief editor of "Encyclopledia Britannica", American philosopher and educator Mortimer J. Adler. That is a subtle programming, or conditioning, of masses and thus patterning of mass psychology. That externally imposed order on our minds is in fact an idiosyncratic way of "killing" time that enslaves us and does nothing for our growth. We become passive observers of other people's lives, instead of designing and living our own. And, take any of the above, there is not a great deal of positive things being reported. The majority of them are sensationalisms, negative and, being played to us hour after hour, day after day (truly, they are no more than a chewing gum for our eyes and our minds), we end up brainwashed, spiritually depersonalised, disorientated, robbed of our own inner experience of importance and responsibility, befooled and programmed to lose the game of life.

Our capability to govern our own destiny has been polluted. As a consequence, our capacity of comprehension and decision-making is rapidly diminishing, our inner values are getting bankrupt, and a state of confusion and difficulties is becoming the archetype of the modern-day life. While many people, easily tempted to join in a mass ritual, tend to flee from this reality via the medium of "entertainment", more and more people seek a quick escape from the environmental hopelessness in drug abuse. And, more and more, our living environment is becoming the polluted environment of the widespread drug trade of epidemic proportions. Yet the problem is in the beliefs about the identity and subsequent behaviour of the users, rather than in drugs themselves.

The power of the drugs resides in the minds of the users who forget that the drugs only remove the symptoms of their problems and not the problems themselves. They look at drugs as "substitute" for feeling and as a "remedy" for alienation and meaningless existence. This "relief" is temporary and it leads to addiction. The adverse consequences of drug abuse range from lowered perception, impaired concentration, tiredness, confused thinking, insensitivity, dulled ability to feel and translate intention into action, altered biochemical reactions in the body, negative emotional reactions lasting many years, through amorality, destroyed relationships, aborted careers, broken families, all the way to the final point – ruined lives. Is there a solution to these? Of course! The surest way to reverse the trend is through education and increased awareness of the population. Those will, in turn, empower the people to become better individuals, physically, mentally and spiritually competent and able to creatively meet the challenges that life brings.

Far too much money is being wasted and many helpless animals tortured and killed in the name of medical research, discovering and trying out new drugs, vaccines, serums, antitoxins, etc. that do not cure, but irritate and harm the body of the user. These medicines, many of which according to Dr John Coleman contain opium – the most addictive substance known, disturb the body of the user in the same way all other stimulants do. Their so-called "therapeutic actions" are in fact reactions of the body against them. After all, how on earth can one expect those substances to cure any disease when the same would actually produce disease if given to a healthy person? Weakened bodies require rest and not interference. The cause of an ailment should be corrected instead of forcing an appearance of health by medicaments. Such an appearance of health is in fact artificial life and a short cut to exhaustion of natural life that ultimately leads to death. Small wonder then, that most of the medical doctors whom I know personally are reluctant to give any medicaments to their own children. So, how much longer will medical professionals continue their experiments before they learn that health cannot be restored by measures that impair it? It seems that they have forgotten, or ignored, the wise words of Nikola Tesla - Serbian-American extraordinary scientist, the ingenious visionary, and beyond question the greatest inventor who ever lived: *"Science is but a perversion of itself unless it has as its ultimate goal the betterment of humanity."*

One more thing: Stop smoking! Cigarettes bring carbon monoxide in your blood instead of oxygen. Nicotine increases your blood pressure, blocks your arteries and consequently makes your heart work faster and harder. People who smoke are more than twice as much risk of heart attack than are people who do not smoke. Tobacco lowers your vitality by 25-50%, reduces your strength and endurance, unsteadies your nerves, impairs hearing and digestion and decreases overall efficiency of your body. It is believed that cigarette paper is impregnated with opium and that it is the main reason for addiction. In the homes of smokers the walls, carpets, furniture, as well as their clothes, hair and skin, become saturated with nicotine poisoning causing the health of those who live there to suffer. You cannot smoke and be healthy. Even most of the smokers that I know think that smoking is bad for the health, but they smoke anyway. What happened to self-honesty and self-respect? Recent scientific studies have concluded that, when you stop smoking, regardless of how much or how long for you have smoked, your risk of heart disease will start to drop, and approximately three years after quitting that risk will decrease dramatically – almost as if you had never smoked. Moreover, statisticians have it that a much greater number of people die from smoking tobacco than from smoking cannabis. Even so, tobacco is not on the list of banned substances. What a hypocrisy!

Tolerated poisoning undermines the body, wastes its nervous energy impairs its functioning and structure, lowers its vital resistance to negative influences and, sooner or later, leads to death.

Governments of developed world are closing their eyes before all this, favouring the big corporate profits before environment conservation and public health. Here I may be accused of standing in a way of progress and called naive for placing my opinion before the masses. So what? I am used to being accused and called worse things than naive. Hey, while my consciousness is in my hands, my reputation is not. Nevertheless, it is the undeniable truth that some of the business enterprises have been based on less than ethical grounds and that the politics of the corporate-state entity, for the sake of the industry and commerce "protection", often suppress and supersede the facts and the right to freedom of expression. I strongly believe that everyone should be in a position to do everything that is required in order to get the results desired – growth, progress, profit, etc. but, <u>without harming anyone in the process</u>.

Chapter Nine

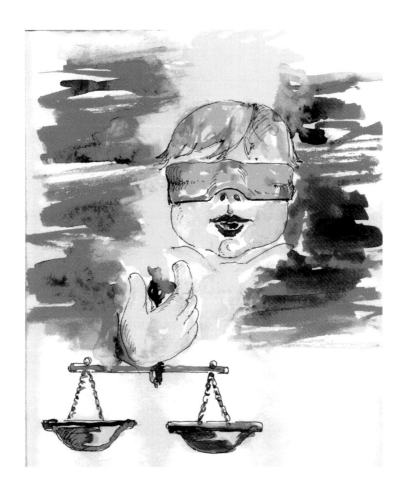

Stress Management

"One word frees us of all the weight and pain of life: that word is Love."

(Sophocles)

STRESS MANAGEMENT

*"One word frees us of all the weight and pain of life: that word is **Love**."* (Sophocles)

For a few years I had been making progress in reversing my crippling condition. Most of my physical needs had been finely tuned and properly met. My body was getting more flexible, the aches were gone and I had considerably higher energy levels. My mind was sharp and my will and self-discipline were sky-high. Yet, I felt something was missing in my inner world.

My drive to act promptly and complete my recovery was slacking. And than, one late evening in January 2004 the lightning struck me. I realised that my emotional and spiritual needs were far from being met. They were "buried" alive, and they were very alive. My self-esteem was somewhat low. And, I did not love myself well enough. What was the cause? I reckon that the pain-killers, which I had been taking, had altered the biochemistry of my body, beclouded my sensibility, and subsequently led to the withdrawal of the feelings.

Those deprived emotional and spiritual needs were bringing a high level of anxiety into my life. The plant deprived of sunshine can never develop fully. The divine power of awareness. That very evening I made a decision to interrupt that pattern and to sort the things out. And I did it decisively and enthusiastically. My list of values got reshuffled. The gift of love became my top priority. On the wings of love, I truly became my own personal challenge. And when I harnessed this unique talent of pure love and blended it with joyful service to others, my life got the new meaning – it became a celebration.

And when I met my soul mate and my mirror – the lady with the radiant glow in her eyes, the sunshine of my life - my light, reflected from that mirror, dispelled my inner weakness and prompted a tremendous

89

transformational odyssey of my being. With honesty, tenderness, goodness and compassion, in place of anxiety, my true self unfolded. My soul went on fire, my spirit soared, my heart – throbbing with joy – began to sing. The scintillating presence of love, joy, peace, happiness and gratitude became the order of the day. And only then, with effortless ease, did I manage to gain back the weight – over 20 kilograms – which I had lost previously. The fruit of love, the miracle of life.

Balance is the key to a harmonious interchange between all of the life domains – spiritual, mental, physical and emotional. Achieving that balance of the inner and the outer world is fundamental for calmness of the spirit, clarity of the mind, health of the body and stability of the emotions. Lack of balance, on the other hand, brings stress and strain to our system and leads to health problems and loss of inner vitality.

"Your health is bound to be affected if, day after day, you say the opposite of what you feel, if you grovel before what you dislike and rejoice at what brings you nothing but misfortune. Your nervous system isn't a fiction; it's a part of your physical body, and your soul exists in space and is inside you, like the teeth in your head. You can't keep violating it with impunity. I found it painful to listen to you, Nicky, when you told us how you were re-educated and grew-up in jail. It was like listening to a circus horse describing how it broke itself in," wrote Boris Pasternak in his famed "Dr. Zhivago".

Our minds have tremendous power over our bodies. Focused mind plays vital part in our health and our life. Almost all our bodily functions are dependant on it: our endocrine system, our emotions, our respiratory, lymphatic and our immune system - our total well-being depends on what we do in our heads. A weakened immune system is a direct consequence of stress, bad physiology and weak focus. Neurosis, anger, fear and other negative emotions are toxins for our body. They are exclusively the result of our reasoning and meanings that we attach to the events in our life. Our thoughts therefore directly affect our bodies. As a matter of fact, almost all illnesses are the consequences of our deluded perceptions. *"The fact that the mind rules the body is, in spite of its neglect by biology and medicine, the most fundamental fact which we know about the process of life,"* said Dr Franz Alexander.

Emotions are pure energy. Their intelligent and balanced expression is beneficial for our health and vitality. But, when they are repressed or expressed in a hysterical manner, vast amounts of vital energy get lost causing essential biochemical changes in the blood and subsequent impairment of our bodily functions. *"Our emotions need to be as educated as our intellect. It is important to know how to feel, how to respond, and how to let life in so that it can touch you,"* articulated it elegantly Jim Rohn.

Contemporary man lives in an age of neurosis and exhaustion. It seems he has conquered the world, but lost himself in the process. His life often feels like a pressure cooker. His energy levels easily get depleted and his immune system often gets weakened. Emotional baggage and old cellular memories create limiting patterns that hold him back from experiencing his full potential. Circa 95% of our thoughts are the same as those of yesterday – distorted old memories that become a lens through which we experience the present. Hence the inner and outer conflicts and confusion in our hearts. There is a great need for a solution that relies on our inner resources to find and maintain balance of our bodily functions.

The way in which we respond to the events in our everyday life can mean the difference between the susceptibility to illness and good health. Stress, which is the result of an unpoised state of mind or more precisely of emotions, invariably weakens our immune system and shortens our life. Most micro-organisms and other disease agents are present in our bodies when we are in sound health and they participate in an illness only when other factors weaken our immune system. People prone to illness are those who feel victims of circumstances, who believe that things just happen to them and that they do not have any influence on their lives. Were they to think that the solutions are within them, the result would be totally different as beyond those circumstances, expectations and past conditioning, which dominate their ordinary attention, lie their intuitive wisdom and creativity.

Emotional overirritation is very common nowadays. Common it may be, but it is not normal. Most of us live tentatively and almost exclusively in our emotions. Internally, it feels like we are drowned in our desires and worries, and enslaved by them. Our emotions greatly affect and often dominate our functions and our life. Invariably, they expend a lot of our vital energy and produce biochemical changes in our bodies. While positive emotions empower us and accelerate our actions, negative emotions on the other hand suspend or even arrest our functioning. The myriad of physical reactions can result from our emotional states. All the more, our lifespan is greatly influenced by them. For these very reasons it is of paramount importance to nurture our emotions. The more ways we know, the broader spectrum of choices we have to respond to our emotions, the richer our life is.

"Stress cooks your brain," an old Chinese proverb has it. Stress is an unspecified response of your being to demands of life. It is nothing else but our interpretation, or judgement, of what is happening to us and as such it creates imbalance in the body. Stress is caused by our polluted attitudes of attachment, grasping (rooted in ignorance), and remorse. Instead of sitting back in times of stress, relaxing and trying to reflect on more creative

ways to cope with challenges of life, influenced by unauthentic needs of our ego and sidetracked by our erroneous projections and fragmented intellectual concepts we tend to stick to one pattern – one that is not producing desired outcomes – and thus get into a loop of negative emotions. Distracted by the tyranny of such appearances and burdened by the self-concern, we consequently lose our awareness of totality, waste our vital energies and greatly diminish our capacities. Therefore, unawareness is the very root of all our neurosis and tensions in a whirlpool of life.

The most destructive of all emotions is fear. It affects the heart, impairs digestion, suspends secretion, nearly paralyses the muscles, greatly wastes your energy and can even cause sudden death. The offsprings of fear such as anger, worry, jealousy, greed, resentment, prejudice, low self-esteem, loneliness, self-pity, grief, anxiety, dishonesty and other negative emotions are nearly as deranging as their mother - fear. However, these negative feelings are only the illusionary creations of your mind and its attitude about the particular event or circumstance. *"Men are disturbed not by things that happen, but by their opinion of the things that happen,"* said Greek philosopher Epictetus. With such awareness and understanding of reality, you can stay unattached, distanced, and respond positively, imaginatively and dynamically to them, and thus arouse more power within yourself that you can use for your own benefit. This very distance breeds freedom. In this way your negative feelings literally defeat themselves, dissolve, evaporate, and you develop a new positive response.

On the other hand, emotions of love, happiness, gratitude, joy, benevolence, cheer, courage, poise, and other positive ones greatly improve your health and vitality and also prolong your life. Bible says: *"A merry heart doeth good like a medicine: but a broken spirit drieth the bones."* It is a great metaphor for how a happy outlook and attitude toward life promote wellbeing, while an unhappy one even suppresses production of blood cells in the bone marrow.

Happiness is our ultimate goal – our life's purpose. It depends on our state of consciousness, on feeling of our self-worth, and is attained by functioning effectively in both our inner and outer world with honesty and dedication to create and grow. When we are aware of our inner destiny, and when we move through life in harmony with that awareness, happiness follows us like a shadow. Happiness is thus a pristine natural state of your being – free from attachments, beliefs, expectations, pretensions, masks, images, projections, clichés, and all other chains and conditioning – unbounded by outer circumstances. Everybody is born happy and everybody is being subtly condemned and made unhappy by the society. If you are not happy right now, here is the reason: misguided by your society's conditioning you have been thinking about what you haven't got in your life, instead of focusing on that which you have got. So, you have to recapture your happiness, your freedom of innocence and intelligence – it is your birthright, it is your responsibility of being your true self. Allow it to manifest in your being by removing the hindrances. It is an adventure, an exploration; it is a blissful journey of self-discovery. Dr Deepak Chopra in his renown book "Quantum Healing" claims that *"At the very instant you think 'I am happy', a chemical messenger translates your emotion, which has no solid existence whatever in the material world, into a bit of matter so perfectly attuned to your desire that literally every cell in your body learns of your happiness and joins in."* And if the expansion of happiness is the ultimate goal, love is its course as well as its main source.

The experience of love in its many forms and ways is beyond a shadow of a doubt the most important factor of exceptional health and vitality. Pure love is the only real miracle-worker, the true nectar of life, the only thing worth living for. The power of the energy of love we humans have available to give one another is remarkable. But, to be able to share it with others you must have it first, you have to love yourself first. If you do not love yourself you cannot love anybody or anything else at all. That is the fact. When you love yourself your ego melts away and your love start overflowing and showering on others. True love understands, forgives and cures. It manifests itself through deep friendship, honesty, devotion, acceptance, respect, trust, compassion, graciousness, patience, creativity, care, goodness, benevolence, tenderness, adoration etc. Love is the highest truth, the ultimate virtue, the supreme good. It is the utmost flowering of consciousness.

Love is the most significant vitamin for the soul. Without the nourishment of love the soul withers away and dies. It is a life-giving force crucial for the sound growth and development of every individual. While infants blessed by the grace of love flourish, lack of love can impair a happy course of an infant's life and even cause his death. And this basic necessity remains with us in our adulthood as well. When the forces greater than yourself seem to overwhelm you, is there anything more reassuring than your beloved holding you tenderly in vibrant watchful silence, or telling you a story or singing you a song? Then you feel being born again, being powerful, being in a land where even angels fear to tread. A blissful web of loving connectedness is a true blaze of glory, a celebration of life, a feeling of being eternal. Being loving and sharing the joy of love with others creates a spontaneous flow of boundless vibrant energy that elevates your soul, cures your mind and revitalises your body. *"Love comforteth like sunshine after rain,"* wrote Shakespeare. Thus, love is much more than a feeling. It is a power – the power of pure awareness and growing understanding of the needs and desires of the self and the significant others in our lives, a power which is spiritual in nature.

Our states of mind, our emotions or sensations alter our feelings and thus profoundly affect our bodies. If an emotion is not translated into constructive action it wastes nerve energy, leads to auto-intoxication and weakens both our mind and body. Therefore, we ourselves create tensions and blocks, and oftentimes we are not even aware of it. When we start identifying ourselves with our thoughts and emotions, our minds become tense and so do our bodies, as they are inseparable parts of a single system. Hence, these tensions and blocks are nothing other than the tightening and contracting of some muscle group of the particular body area linked to discharge of particular emotion. Only once we become aware of this fact, only once our awareness takes us away from our minds, can we start releasing the tensions and dissolving the blocks. Fully aware, we need to open ourselves to the impulses and emotions which are buried alive underneath the muscular cramp, run them through tense area of the body and release them. Then only will our bodies start relaxing. Freedom to feel and express our emotions brings a sense of harmony to us. Self-discipline is thus necessary for refinement of emotions, transformation of stress and anxiety into awareness, and accomplishment of the spirit of sound mind and sound life.

While tensions waste our energies, relaxation (mind at rest; letting go) conserves and replenishes them. Many techniques can help us to dissolve our tensions, restore balance and experience the flow of our creative energy. An experience of balance is achievable through the practice of meditation.

Meditation turns our awareness deep within ourselves, brings an incredible sense of connection and a profound realisation that our most intimate self is universal in nature and enables us to find that balance in all the facets of our experience of life. It is an experience that we have and nurture rather than something that we do with our minds and our emotions. Awareness, transcending all distractions of time, space, matter and energy, supersedes our intellect and our senses. Ultimately, it clears the debris of our tensions and leads us to an expanded understanding of our true nature, of who we really are. Perfectly balanced and fully in charge of our minds and emotions we are able to unleash our potential further and face each situation with grace, inner peace and wisdom.

Like any other skill, meditation takes practice, discipline and diligence to learn. Begin by lying flat or sitting comfortably and paying attention to your breathing. Inhale slowly through your nose and let your breath expand your chest and abdomen as your diaphragm drops. As the breath rhythmically fills you and flows out, you slowly withdraw your attention from the external world and bring your awareness inside. Let go of your mind and a sense of deep relaxation will follow. Witness your floating thoughts, but do not follow them, go beyond your mind, remain aware of your breathing, and a clarity will arise. This conscious breathing combined with perfect alertness clears all tensions, develops the flow of energy throughout our body and brings us a feeling of inner peace, vitality and integrity – virtual unity of the whole universe. Practised over time, meditation enables us to awaken, absorb all experiences deeply within ourselves, sail through our life relaxed and grow free of limitations.

Relaxation through awareness is the foundation of the sound internal strength. To this should be added the development of our emotional, spiritual, mental and physical capacities the greatest proportion of which remains untapped throughout our lives. World-renown

Scottish psychiatrist, Ronald D. Laing emphasised this beautifully: *"We think much less than what we know, we know much less than we love, we love much less than there is, and to this precise extent we are much less than what we are."* Doesn't this blow your mind up? The only peace and joy in life lie in the pursuit and actualisation of this unrealised unlimited potential lying dormant within you – the true wonder of you. It has been said that most of us die before we are fully born. Do not let that happen to you, please.

Apart from learning meditation as the ultimate relaxation technique, there are some other things you should pay attention to. To start with, learn to prioritise your schedule and do the most important things first. Then, stop trying to adjust the reality to your ideas and images about it and accept it as it is – accept yourself, respect yourself and love yourself. Do not burden yourself by the past or worry too much about the future. Learn from your past and plan for the future, but – live in the here and now, the present moment, the only true life there is. If you are concerned over something, discuss it with someone whom you really trust. Try to simplify your life by eliminating trivia, so that you can experience more of the essential life. Remember: your ego may be a great technician, but is not creative; let go of it. Be aware of your communication, as it is the most crucial factor that determines your relationships to others and to yourself – be consistent in what you think, say and do. See people for what they truly are, as whole and innocent – stop judging and criticising. Meet your need to feel fulfilment through accepting, loving, sharing and giving unconditionally. And, whenever your heart calls for it, seek contentment in solitude – the only freedom from the crowd, freedom from the other, freedom from attachment. In that solitude drop forgetfulness and find yourself – move out of your personality, which is your gift from the crowd, let it disperse, and remember yourself. Drop your need to be needed – it is an ego need – attain a crystallized soul and remember who you truly are. When you summon the courage to be solitary, in that freedom you will grow in detachment, your body and soul will get integrated, you will grow in joy and you will become healthier.

Life is precious. When it brings you too many challenges, demands, options, you become anxious. When there are too few of these, you get bored. Sounds like inner civil war, doesn't it? Your mind and your soul get confused. Yet, inner peace is within your grasp. Inner order is attainable when you live a life of contemplated action guided by your inner wisdom and truth. If you find your life's purpose and pursue it with a great resolve, all your thoughts, feelings and activities will be congruent with one another and, ultimately, harmony will come to your consciousness. Your psychic energy will always be usefully employed, regardless of what is happening to you. This potent threesome – purpose, resolve and harmony – unify life and give it meaning, so that every living moment makes sense and is enjoyable.

Sensibly chose to live an interesting and exciting life, live life in wonder and awe, create vibrant physical states and see for yourself how it affects your health and vitality. *"If a name be needed, let the name be wonder, and then from wonder to wonder, existence opens,"* said ancient Chinese sage Lao Tzu. Yes, it does take time, patience, persistence, sympathetic understanding, re-education and most importantly toxin elimination through observing the natural laws of life, but it is doable.

Nourish your soul, nourish your mind, nourish your self-esteem. Malnutrition in these areas leads to suffering. Whether you are healthy or in pain, it is a reflection of your state of mind, a reflection of the quality of your attention. Whichever kind of emotional energy your mind creates, it gets translated in the corresponding state of your physical body. Well-balanced mental diet is the pillar of your well-being.

Medical, psychological, biological and social sciences all confirm the beneficial effects of friendly emotions upon our health and vitality. And yet, our ignoble practices are in great discord with our knowledge. As Ralph Waldo Emerson once said: *"The measure of mental health is the disposition to find good everywhere."*

To be in charge of your outer life you have to be in charge of your inner life, as the outer is the reflection of the inner. Striving after the unauthentic needs of your inflated ego brings misery to your life because along the way you might capture all the riches of the world but you will lose your soul and feel empty. Only by going beyond your thoughts and your feelings, only by becoming silent and bringing awareness to your experiences, can you reach the very core of your authentic being – that which is free from all society's conditioning and chains, that which can give you back the authorship of your life, that which is your only true guide to blissful harmonious existence – your spirit. Harness its power, stay centred and focus on loving, growing and sharing rather than feeling good in a moment. It is up to you to decide in which direction you prefer to travel. Knowing which is the right direction to take is wisdom. Taking it is integrity. The choice is yours. Choose well and take full responsibility for it.

Now, you are prepared to learn the art of...

Chapter Ten

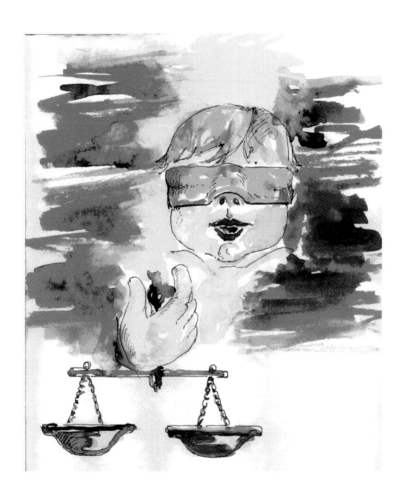

Change Initiation

"You are what your deep, driving desire is.
As your desire is, so is your will.
As your will is, so is your deed.
As your deed is, so is your destiny."

(Brihadaranyaka Upanishad IV.4.5)

CHANGE INITIATION

"You are what your deep, driving desire is.
As your desire is, so is your will.
As your will is, so is your deed.
As your deed is, so is your destiny."
(Brihadaranyaka Upanishad IV.4.5)

The principles explained in preceding chapters could make a startling difference in how you view the world and how the world views you. They are not the theories to be enforced on your life, not at all. They are the universal living truths engraved upon your timeless heart. If only you would listen to it.

Just remain true to life and see the ill effects of your living against life undone. Hey, do not take my word at face value - become aware of it, try to understand it clearly, adopt the correct view of reality, take what is right for you, experience it, and convince yourself. It is much easier than you think it may be. Nevertheless, not many people do it. Do you find yourself rushing around from the moment you get up in the morning until the minute you go to sleep at night? If you have followed me thus far, I am sure you do not want to be in that category any more. You will have made a decision. If so, I congratulate you. You are ready to take charge of your health, your vitality and your life.

Let me ask you yet another question: Which direction are you heading in on your current life track? Whichever it is, please be responsible human being and take the choices right for you, plan according to your needs rather than live life according to someone else's plan for you, and recognise and accept the fact that there are the laws of Nature concerning us all.

With regards to the above, I am sure you have been making the best choices from those health concerning choices you have been aware of. Maybe you simply did not have enough choices. Here, you have been presented with some illuminating insights, some revealing facts, some enlightening possibilities – possibilities that will empower you to respond to the same situations in a different way and achieve totally different results. I myself take no credit for their invention or novelty (they have existed as long as human life on Earth has), other than their recognition and attempt to instil them into your awareness so as to enable you to take a decisive action.

Awareness is the seed of change. By posing new choices, it awakens your inner wisdom that questions and helps you tame your habitual reactions. More often than not, your mind is dominated by the thoughts you habitually feed it with. Stop that. Surrender to the awareness of the illusions of your mind, of your desires, your fears and your habits. Let the new insights start arising, develop deeper understanding and wisely take charge over the factors that govern your health and vitality. To the increased awareness your whole being will spontaneously respond and consequently your life will unfold.

Now, commit to making some new resolutions and make a plan for conforming your life to the laws of Mother Nature. Accept the highest possible standard. Then, with total immersion, take action and follow your plan. If you do not succeed outright, stay alert, open up to the wisdom of Nature, be flexible, identify barriers and try again with a new approach. Along the way, have confidence in yourself about embarking on a new healthy behaviour and make sure your resolution has meaning to you. Do not force things, as effort almost always leads to inner conflict. Intelligently resort to awareness of reality instead. This faithful and persistent employment of your awareness builds an unstoppable momentum that, in a quantum leap, turns your burning desires into reality.

Attempting to make a profound change can be risky – you might say. And I agree with you. We risk being controversial, misunderstood, lonely and wrong. To change, we must take those risks, or there will be no change. Doing what is right is more important than worrying about who is right, isn't it? Other's opinions cannot be more important than you, than the splendour of your existence – inexhaustible, unfathomable, unrepeatable. Still frightened? Well, that's what freedom is like. It calls to be taken. Herbert Otto said: *"Change and growth take place when a person has risked himself and dares to become involved with experimenting with his own life."*

On the other hand, your attachments to anything and anyone are standing in a way of change. Those attachments are just the food for your mind, for your ego. They absorb energy from your body and create habits. Then your habits become your very nature and your nature becomes secondary. And then you end up living through your habits, or better said: your past habits live through you, draining your energy, and – you become their slave.

Lasting change means being prepared to make some habit sacrifices. Know clearly what your new attitude can bring to your life and what you would lose by not adopting a healthier practice. And the beauty of it all is that once you approach a new idea with active openness and subtle receptivity, you do not need to think consciously about the change – it will happen to you, it will manifest through you. Your awareness of the truth will stir your intuition and lead to the change. It is like sowing a seed in a fertile soil. As it sprouts, it grows larger and larger...and it blossoms... How surprised will you be? Employed over the period of time, this new discipline born out of awareness will become a refined behaviour of choice, a part of your realized potentiality and your life.

In summary, achieving and maintaining your health and vitality means changing your attitude and your relationship to yourself first and then to others and everything else that we have talked about in this book. Only that which you are aware of and understand can you change. Awareness is your only path to change. Unify the practical information presented hereby with your intuitive wisdom and experience the transformation. Change and growth are the end result of all true learning and merging of awareness, understanding and action. The law of Nature will either reward you or penalise you, according to the life you live.

Here, I would like to cite Sam Levinson's dictum: *"If you don't change, I'll come and get you!"*

A famous poem says that you are the master of your fate and the captain of your soul. It is all up to you. You know the benefits of change. Also, you are the only person who knows who is going to lose out if you do not awaken and initiate the change. Do not wait. The time to start is right now, as just a tiny stretch away is a living fire of your unlimited potential. Go ahead - unleash it! Let go of the past, let go of your guilt, let go of your ego-grasping neurotic mind. *"Wisdom is to speak the truth and act in keeping with its nature,"* wrote Heraclitus. Use your imagination, follow the ageless wisdom of Nature and Truth with zeal, zest, and profound sense of certainty and – enjoy the journey.

Remember: <u>if you believe in yourself, you will be unstoppable, and you will live the dreams that you hold quietly in your heart and soul.</u>

Epilogue

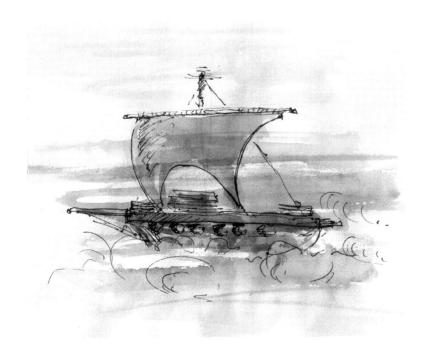

"A journey of a thousand miles
begins with a single step."
(Confucious)

"There are no incurable diseases, only incurable people."

(Bernie Siegel)

EPILOGUE

"There are no incurable diseases, only incurable people."
(Bernie Siegel)

This book is a reminder that nothing in life matters more than health and vitality. When you are healthy and vital nothing you desire is beyond your reach. On the other hand, you can have money and everything else, if you are not healthy all that matters very little.

Hypnosis of social conditioning prevents us from paying conscious attention to our natural bodily functions. To reinforce our reality we seek a feedback from what our environment defines as "normal" and therefore "real". Influenced by our parents, educators, priests, politicians, and the commercial broadcasting lies, we easily and readily conform to social "demands" and become stereotypes. We consume our foods in the customary way, drink what is trendy, smoke to be "cool", buy the popular magazines and books, and so on. By blindly following the "fashion", we loose our uniqueness, our individuality, and become slaves to new gimmicks. Left to run on an automatic pilot we are unable to cope well with the effects of either autointoxication or external agents, which trouble our immune system. The flow of our energy and inner intelligence becomes compromised and as a result our bodies deteriorate. *"Man does not die; he kills himself,"* an ancient sage said. And, indeed, modern man is engaged in committing a slow suicide often without even being consciously aware of it.

I am going to say this again, although I am sure you already know it – as it is easy to do these things you read about in this book, it is also easy not to do them. Let me be impolite enough to ask you the same old question one more time: Is there anything in your life more important to you than your health and vitality? I do not think so. Without good health it is difficult to enjoy what life has to offer. I am sure you already know this simple truth, and yet many of you take your health and vitality for granted as more pressing matters like money, status, hobbies, family commitments, etc. take over. And only when troubles start to show do we notice and begin to fight back. From there on, only a profound change in your lifestyle can bring desired results. Nothing else. To believe otherwise would be foolish.

In order to improve your health and vitality you must attain independence of your mind, expand your awareness, let your perceptions crystallize, set your spirit free, and start acting intelligently. That transformation can begin in an instant. All it requires is your decision to do something about it, and than to take action and do it regardless of what else may come your way. Instead of beating yourself with "Why me, Lord?" ask the questions that will empower you, like " What can I learn from this?" or "How can I turn the things around?" The answer is usually very simple, especially if you truly care and are willing to assume the responsibility. Start by focusing on changing those deep-rooted habits, wrong habits of thought, that put your health and vitality in jeopardy, and give your organism a chance to recuperate its dissipated vital energy. To turn this awareness into action, and ultimately into your life-style, you need a little discipline. Let the disciplined effort of doing what is right wipe away the effects of ignorance and neglect. Let your actions, born out of awareness, guide and shape your thinking habits.

The benefits of simple, subtle habit change will accomplish dramatic results and probably extend your life. Please always keep in mind that your habits do reveal your character and also that your character traits without awareness are just pretensions that enslave you. Only people who live without consciousness need a character – it is only a crutch. Have courage to explore the joys of your consciousness rather than stay confined to any habit. Your life is being transformed with the expansion of your consciousness. Undoubtedly, detached, compassionate consciousness is an awesome healing force.

"Learning is nothing but remembering," said Socrates. It is an awakening of wisdom that already exists within you. I have reminded you of some simple facts of life to help you along that voyage of change, or attitude engineering if you prefer, and encourage you to give those things to yourself – they are **your birthright**. Unless they are integrated and constructively used, nothing will happen. And with passage of time you may even forget how to use them. There is an old adage which says: *"To be is to do."* Action follows being – it springs spontaneously out of your being. For a new discipline to be learned, it must be tried out. So, what are you waiting for? Go on, make that decision, commit yourself to turning the experience around, let your intuition be your guide and your teacher, put yourself on the line, and transform your health and vitality forever. Do it now!

This book has been no more than what was intended – to be a sharing, the sharing of my experience and reflection on the insights gained along the path to regaining my health and vitality. Whether its message – message of freedom through awareness and understanding – is received or not, writing it has been worth the effort. It has been a wonderful gift to myself – the gift that I share with you. For myself, I truly live what I preach here. The mantle is firmly in your hands now. As Nikos Kazanstakis, a flamboyant Greek novelist and philosopher, said: *"You have your brush and colours, paint paradise, and in you go."*

In closing, I want to thank you for staying with me this long. May the time and effort you spent reading this book be rewarded with what you become aware of by it. My final message to you is:

Live healthy, live happy, live long...and remember: <u>the road to exceptional health and vitality is always under construction</u>.

*"Everything in the universe
is within you.
Ask all from yourself."*

(Rumi)

৯৹৵

*"It is only with the heart
that one can see rightly;
what is essential
is invisible to the eye."*

(Antoine de Saint-Exupéry)

ABOUT THE AUTHOR

Milorad Masic is an up-and-coming wellness educator and coach whose "secrets" of exceptional health and vitality have already helped many people from different walks of life.

He was born and raised in Serbia where, after graduating from university in Belgrade, he first became a Geography lecturer. His subsequent wish to seek wider horizons has taken him on a worldwide journey of self-discovery.

Several years ago, while tirelessly traversing the new paths, disaster struck. Pain-killers that had been prescribed to cure his severe arthritic condition almost killed him. His stomach collapsed, he rapidly lost a lot of weight, and almost lost his life. Only a strong will and a determination to find his own solutions to this life-debilitating illness kept him going.

The years that followed were in his own words: 'The years of my search for lost treasure – the exceptional health and vitality which is the birthright of us all.'

In *Your Birthright* Milorad shares with us the empowering message about the fundamental laws and principles of healthy and vital life – often neglected by the majority of us and unacknowledged by modern-day conventional medicine – on a mission to help us attain awareness of what he feels are life's greatest values.

Currently he lives in London where he is working on his second book.